ON THE SCENT

Unlocking the
mysteries of smell
– and how its loss can
change your world

SCENT

PAOLA TOTARO & ROBERT WAINWRIGHT

Elliott&Thompson

First published 2022 by
Elliott and Thompson Limited
2 John Street
London WC1N 2ES
www.eandtbooks.com

ISBN: 978-1-78396-642-4

Picture Credits:
Page 283: Shutterstock.com

9 8 7 6 5 4 3 2 1

A catalogue record for this book is available from
the British Library.

Typesetting: Marie Doherty
Printed by CPI Group (UK) Ltd, Croydon, CR0 4YY

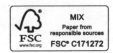

To the world's olfactory scientists, physicians and researchers — past, present and future — whose passion and persistence contributes immeasurably to human health.

Contents

PART 3

Foreword

I fell ill without warning. Four days of lungs on fire then, as quickly as the searing pain had come, it went – and with it my sense of smell and taste.

I remember vividly the moment I first noticed its absence. I had been washing my hands for what felt like the hundredth time when the moisturising lotion I use – a potent mix of mandarin rind, cedar atlas and rosemary leaf – yielded nothing, not even the hint of a fragrance. Confused, I uncapped and sniffed several of my perfumes, each one ever more desperately. *Nada.*

Panicked, I scrabbled in the cupboard for a floral, ammonia-based toilet cleaner that normally makes you pull back in shock when you remove the cap but even when I buried my nose in the neck of the bottle, still nothing. The sensory vacuum was so intense that for a few seconds I felt as if I were in free-fall in a faulty elevator.

The UK had been in first lockdown for less than a week but that night, 27 March 2020, Prime Minister Boris Johnson confirmed he was isolating in Number 10 Downing Street after testing positive for Covid-19. In the United States, a visibly tearful Joe Biden empathised on television with those unable to visit loved ones critically ill with the new virus.

Convinced my absence of smell could only be the dreaded Covid, I ignored my GP's perfunctory dismissal of the symptom by telephone and decided to self-isolate. Less than a fortnight earlier my (co-author) husband and I had returned to London after hiking Hadrian's Wall, crossing England west to east, in five days. It was a marathon walk of more than 16 miles each day, battling 60-mile-an-hour winds and more icy mud and rain than I care to remember. We'd come back feeling elated and fit but now feared the unknown.

Locked in my frightening sensory desert in those first dark days, I began to Google the loss of smell. I learned it is called anosmia if you lose it completely, hyposmia when it is partial, and that congestion and inflammation sparked by viral illnesses such as the common cold are the most common culprits. The strange thing for me was that my nose did not feel stuffy and I could breathe without impediment but as the air entered it felt as if I'd inhaled dry ice deep into my nasal cavity and the frozen wafts then speared directly into my brain.

I would find out much later that this was exactly the time that Google and other search engines registered a global surge in requests for information on 'loss of smell' as hundreds of thousands of others in the same position as me scrambled to understand what was happening to them. In some ways, I was fortunate because I had been immersed in reporting the earliest days of the Covid crisis in northern Italy and had been intrigued by an increasing flurry of anecdotal reports from physicians in the worst hit region of Lombardy about the sudden onset of anosmia in patients testing positive for the virus. My brother, an intensive-care specialist running one of Australia's biggest public-hospital ICU units in Sydney, alerted me to similar, informal reports from South Korea and Germany and agreed I should presume Covid infection and isolate. Most mornings, my inbox would ping with links and reports he was hearing about the phenomenon from his own clinical networks.

Fascinated by the apparent vacuum in scientific or medical understanding of what was unfolding, I trawled news, science and medical sites daily, searching Twitter and other social-media discussion for any mention of this strange and sudden syndrome. I was not alone in this either: the sheer volume of web chatter combined with clinicians sharing experiences from the coalface in their surgeries and hospitals had also caught the attention of chemosensory scientists around the world.

※

Amid the chaos of the first lockdown and the early quest for information, it dawned on me that the loss of my fifth sense was not only weighing heavily but had begun to feel more and more like an amputation. A part of me seemed to be missing, and the more time passed, the more I was mourning its loss. I have always been hypersensitive to smells, able to tell when my children had been in a smoky room, quick to identify fragrances worn by others and inordinately disturbed by lingering cooking smells in the house. My visual memory is deeply wired to smell and some of the most important moments in my life – both happy and sad – are indelibly interlinked with olfactory experiences. I still associate the fleeting childhood anxiety associated with my mother preparing to go out for an evening heralded by a spritz of a particular Christian Dior perfume. And most of us who have become parents ourselves share the universal joy of the immediately familiar scent of our newborn baby's head.

As I was forced to consider the role of smell in my life, I realised too that I often referred to olfactory impressions in my work as a foreign correspondent. During one particularly hot summer just before the Arab Spring, I'd spent a week with the Italian coast-guard patrolling the seas between Libya and the tiny rocky island of Lampedusa, the closest landfall to Italy. More and more people were risking their lives to flee Africa by sea in a bid to forge new lives in Europe, and while I witnessed several, terrifying mid-sea rescues, one in particular had remained with me. My magazine feature opened with the overwhelming 'stench of fear mingled with acrid sweat' as scores of terrified young men were hauled from the rapidly sinking fishing boat onto the safety of the coastguard's launch.

Hiking the foothills of the Himalayas to document the work of an ophthalmic surgeon who removed cataracts to return sight to blind villagers in remote mountain communities, it was the bitter smell of antiseptic wiped around patients' eyes that remained with me. Similarly, in Kathmandu's Pashupatinath Temple, Nepal's oldest Hindu site, the pungent oily smoke from the human funeral pyres, and the morbid beauty of the stinking swirl around them, struck me even more than the sound of raw grief lancing the silence. When Covid struck, I'd just embarked on my PhD and found myself in the bizarre situation of writing and researching a book about a pioneering French perfumer in nineteenth-century Naples who launched a line of prestigious, highly fragrant soaps made with olive oil, not animal fats – while having no sense of smell of my own. (His story was of particular interest to me as he was my great-great-grandfather.)

Now, locked down at home in London, I could smell nothing of my domestic world either, which made life feel alien and flat. In normal times, walking the dog each day is a stop–start affair (much to my husband's irritation) because I revel in slowing down and inhaling the smell of the outdoors, whether it is freshly mown grass, the heady scent of cherry blossom, new eruptions of daffodils or the first sprigs of climbing rose. Flowers without scent felt like a cruel mockery, their beauty visible but lacking the dimension I love most.

As the weeks passed, it felt wrong to complain when so many were critically ill or dying but the few pleasures left during lockdown – food, booze, the outdoors – had lost their joy. At the dinner table, red wine tasted like salty water, white wine like a mild, odourless vinegar. My favourite aperitif, gin, was barely perceptible in the overwhelming, cloying sweetness of the tonic. Steak felt like biting into a slab of flabby leather, chicken a horrifying, bony, rubber, while dark chocolate, my favourite, tasted like unscented soap.

Appalled but also journalistically intrigued, I continued to look into the mechanisms behind our senses of taste and smell. I learned that while the process of tasting starts when we chew and grind our food down with our teeth, true flavour comes from the chemical mix of odours released as we do so. The tongue perceives five basic tastes – salt, sweet, sour, umami (savoury), bitter. But as we consume say, a delicious lemon tart, the zingy citrus molecules are let loose inside our mouths to mix with sweet, buttery pastry and, as we swallow, this symphony of odours is shunted upward through the back of the throat and into the nasal passage for processing by our olfactory neurones and brain.

This is called retronasal olfaction: it is different from the process known as orthonasal olfaction, which occurs whenever we simply put our noses to a smell and sniff. It's an interesting process to put to the test: blindfold a friend and ensure they hold their nose so they can breathe only through their mouth. Cut up and peel two fruits of similar texture, perhaps an apple and not too ripe pear or melon and firm mango, then ask them to identify what they are eating. Without retronasal smelling, they will be unable to differentiate between the two.

As the weeks passed, I found this pall of blandness made me search for texture as if somehow adding a mix of consistencies in food could make up for their lack of taste. Crunchy, crisp foods provided some relief from the monotony, as did creamy cheeses or velvety soups if eaten with hard crackers or toasted bread. My nose, brain and mouth seemed to be desperate for new signposts to navigate food and make it palatable. It turned out that I wasn't alone in the need for texture and that this is a common response in those who have lost smell: the creator of the now ubiquitous Ben and Jerry's ice-cream brand, Ben Cohen, was born anosmic and his instinctive desire to add new 'bits' to his ice-cream – chocolate chips, cookies, dough – to make up for the absence of smell and taste made him a millionaire.

Smell and taste are, of course, inextricably linked. They are also the least understood of our senses. Our sensory reading of the world is the product of layers of learning and association, which then work hand in hand with a series of intricate neurological responses. Naturally, we imagine our senses working together, a harmony between sight, hearing, touch and smell, even though we may not be generally aware of the process. But when you put your nose to something to smell it and, suddenly, the resulting sensation bears no relationship to what you expected, the effect is not only startling but jolts you to a conscious awareness of the disrupted sense.

As I entered the sixth month, to my elation, my sense of smell began to return, at times fleeting and often barely perceptible. Then I began to notice strange effects with no apparent cause. I would become overwhelmed by a smell of firewood smoke or burning rubber. I learned that these olfactory disturbances are known to clinicians as parosmia when existing smells are distorted and phantosmia when smells are hallucinated or conjured out of nowhere. Recognised as occurring in the wake of viral illnesses such as colds or traumatic brain injury, before Covid they were relatively rare, little understood and usually the province of ear and nose specialists. I was lucky because my nose perceived an odd, sweet baking smell even in things from which you would normally recoil, like a dog poo bag. Hundreds and thousands of others have not been as fortunate, their food, coffee, even tap water haunted by overpowering smells of sewage or rotting garbage. It would be many months before a flavour scientist and a philosopher would combine their knowledge to explain to me how and why recovering from anosmia can throw you into confusion between fair and foul.

The late, great neuroscientist and writer Oliver Sacks wrote eloquently about many of these strange syndromes three decades ago: the loss experienced by patients who had lost their sense of smell; the terror and distress of phantosmia. He introduced us to a woman transfixed by grief when she couldn't recognise the smell of her own baby; a man's faltering explanation of the deadening effect of anosmia on lovemaking; and a passionate home cook who could not enjoy the tantalising smell of onions frying – or of her pots burning on the stove.

But he also showed how the loss of one sense can sometimes highlight the liminal space between the others, telling the story of an anosmic who could smell the scent of a flower but only when he could gaze at it, or the patient who knew that the smell of a phantom roast beef cooking was the warning that a migraine was about to hit. Only a few years ago these were stories of the weird and wonderful. Today, millions of people worldwide have experienced the abrupt loss of their fifth sense, with many later forced to wrestle with a plethora of distressing distortions of their ability to smell.

The unimaginable speed and collaborative nature of the scientific effort needed to develop a vaccine and inoculate entire nations has already been likened to the Apollo moon missions and will be seen as one of modern history's greatest medical and scientific achievements. But behind this enormous accomplishment lies another equally exciting medical detective story, one that saw an eclectic group of researchers, among them chemosensory scientists and clinicians, philosophers and psychologists, anosmia sufferers and their advocates, band together, set aside rivalries and explore and unveil some of the greatest mysteries surrounding the sense of smell.

Come with me on a journey of olfactory discovery. Meet many of the world's leading experts, wonder at the science and hear the stories of the many patients who forged a path back to life and health in the wake of the Covid pandemic.

PART 1

1

The Story of O(lfaction)

From the moment we take our first breath, we inhale and exhale around 22,000 times a day, flooding our olfactory system with a panoply of odours in the instant before our lungs fill with air. The outside world can tell us immediately if our room smells musty or our clothes need a wash; if the baby's nappy needs changing or the jasmine outside is in bloom at last. Some odours, like a wet, muddy dog, are immediately identifiable (how I missed this during my year of anosmia!) while others, like the smell of your own house, are barely perceptible and register only if we think specifically about them or something has changed. We can recognise a friend's perfume as floral or woody, differentiate between strawberries ripening in a bowl and the bananas turning brown beside them, recognise the unshakeable reek of stale cigarette smoke in a teenager's jacket or the zing of orange zest as it is grated into a bowl.

What we perceive as a single odour is, however, often a mix of hundreds of different chemicals – the 400 individual receptors in the nose recognise and differentiate between a vast number of compounds. When the smell of frying onions permeates your

3

house, specific receptors detect components of the odour and lead you to the kitchen. But the relationship between the number of receptors that we have and the number of odorants we can identify remains mysterious. How they behave, at times, can be equally odd. The scent of violets, for example, used as a cure for headache in ancient times, much loved by Napoleon and highly fashionable in the Victorian period, is produced by a group of chemical compounds known as ionones. Violet is sweet, soft and even a little powdery. I love it very much because my grandfather always picked a small bunch for my grandmother as soon as they emerged in the earliest, still chilly days of spring. While the posy smelled glorious at first, it also seemed quite hard to 'catch' and retain the fragrance – violet scent is known for this ephemeral quality. The ionones, which stimulate our olfactory receptors and bind to them, can behave quite oddly as they can also temporarily shut off our perception of the scent. You can sniff as hard as you can but you won't get any more smell or intensity from the violet. Perfumers know to be sparing with ionones. It's not that you've lost your sense of smell; it is the pesky yet fragrant ionones desensitising your nose to a perfume.

◈

Smell is the most ancient of our senses, honed by millions of years of evolution and crucial to all forms of life on earth. Careful sensing of the environment is key to animal and human reproduction and survival, protecting against unseen dangers such as toxic foods and gases, smoke and fire.

For a long time, it was thought that olfaction existed only among more complex organisms and that it evolved with animals on land. Scientists now know that the oldest living organisms – bacteria and single-cell animals – had also developed ways to detect the chemical composition of their surroundings. In 2010, a team of marine microbiologists at Newcastle University in the UK became the first to show that primeval organisms have 'noses' and can detect the presence of nutrients (or rivals) through the sense of smell. When bacteria were exposed to ammonia, a source of nitrogen needed for their growth and reproduction, they competed and joined forces to get closer to it, creating a kind of biofilm along the way.[1] This behaviour provides us with a vivid glimpse into the evolutionary process and how the earliest living creatures learned to navigate their environment through smell, using it to find what they need to grow and compete with each other. Many other single-cell organisms, including yeasts and slime moulds, have also now been shown to use a form of 'smell' to navigate their surroundings.

The mechanisms involved in olfaction are, of course, vastly different depending on the life form. We vertebrates use our noses to draw odour molecules into the body and up to the brain; insects and crustaceans use their antennae; while molluscs and soft-bodied animals such as worms and snails have developed specific nerve cells in their heads that perform an olfactory function.

The intricacy and complexity of this evolution is illustrated by what unfolds inside the human nose (see page 283). Every time we draw breath, we inhale airborne particles, including odorant molecules, from the vast sea of gases that surround us. As these odorants enter the nasal cavity, they pass along bony ridges – turbinates – that are covered in soft tissue and mucus. These swell and increase blood flow, acting a little like an air-conditioning unit to retain moisture and warmth and stop dust particles from entering our lungs. At the same time, tiny hairlike projections called cilia help move odour molecules onward and upward into the olfactory epithelium – a thin, yellowish layer of tissue no bigger than a postage stamp at the very top of the nasal cavity – where they dissolve. The epithelium is lined with receptors, the highly specialised cells that transmit information to the olfactory bulb, located at the front of the brain, above the nasal cavity. We humans have millions of these receptors but only 400 different receptor-cell types and while we now know the mechanisms that bring odours from the outside world into the brain for processing, exactly how we identify and distinguish between the estimated trillion odours that scent our world remains shrouded in mystery.

When I was first grappling with my loss of smell, I found it both fascinating and unbelievable that we can land a spaceship safely on Mars, analyse and photograph the red planet's surface, and yet we still don't quite understand how and why things smell the way they do.

Two and a half thousand years ago, the materialist philosophers of ancient Greece argued that atoms were the basic building blocks of all matter – including odour – and ascribed them particular shapes. Bitter, sharp smells were thought to be made of pointy atoms, perhaps because they can make us physically wince with discomfort, while pleasant fragrances and scents were imagined as round, soft and gently curved atoms.

As it turns out, relatively recent studies on insects have demonstrated that there is a relationship of sorts between the structure of some odour molecules and how some receptors respond to them. However, a lock-and-key theory, which suggests that some smells act like keys, unlocking specific receptors, has now been shown to be impossible as with just 400 keys to a trillion or so locks,[2] the maths just doesn't stack up. In fact, science has revealed that some receptor cells respond only to very specific types of odour molecules while others are more broadly tuned – what researchers quaintly describe as 'promiscuous' because they react to so many different molecules.

Philosopher and cognitive scientist Professor Ann-Sophie Barwich likens the way receptors and odorants work together to the tango. Dancing with one particular partner, she says, can lead to a very special kind of erotic tension that might not be felt with someone else. And partnership with another dancer might make you think, 'Oh please, never again.' Smell is as fickle and as complicated: olfactory receptors can be attracted to a particular smell, reject it or respond openly to several aspects of yet another smell.

Professor Barry Smith, also a philosopher and founder of the University of London's Centre for the Study of the Senses, suggested I try to understand the process by conjuring a familiar smell, perhaps a rose, cut grass or milk that's gone off:

> We know that each receptor codes for many different odours at the same time – roses, cut grass, sour milk – but each odour molecule is coded by many receptors. None of these smells has a direct receptor match; they have many-to-many matches, not one-to-one.
>
> Imagine that you've got benzaldehyde, which is a single-molecule odour and yet its smell is also ambiguous. If you give it to one person, they will tell you it smells of marzipan while someone else will tell you it smells like maraschino

cherries. In smell, there is no nice strict relationship as occurs with primary colours or musical scales.

If that isn't messy enough, it gets even more mysterious when it comes to odour mixtures. Sometimes when you mix two smells together, you can still recognise each separately – chocolate and orange that have been combined into a pudding, for example.

But there are other smells that end up creating something entirely new when combined. Vanilla and strawberry mixed up create an odd, indistinguishable sweetish new odour. This is how perfumers develop new scents, experimenting with different odour solutions and combining them in varying strengths until the primary ingredient stops being the dominant one and a distinct new fragrance is formed. Perfumers call this an accord (the French word for a chord) as it is similar to the way you hold down several notes in music to create a unique sound. Some odorants have been found to actively suppress a secondary scent while others can enhance their partner, significantly changing the fragrance of the final product.

Professor Smith noted that wine is another good example as it contains esters, the organic acids that occur during fermentation and give your glass that fruity aroma. When you add dimethyl sulphide in the right proportion it boosts the wine's fruitier notes. But if you just keep increasing it, suddenly the wine will smell awful, like rotten eggs. 'Wine making, perfumery . . . odour chemistry really is puzzling,' says Professor Smith.

While we know about the myriad smell 'signatures', we don't know exactly how they are processed and decoded by the brain to form a recognisable smell. The tango is a good analogy here too.

Dancers will move between moments when one will be dominant and lead the other – a dynamic smell receptors go through too. One might be uppermost and force a molecule to bend a little to activate and turn it on, while a completely different smell mix might act like a turn-off, dampening receptor activity. This smell ballet can unfold countless times in each of the 400 receptors in the nose as their reactions are sent back to the brain for processing. Scientists call these complex patterns of activity in our olfactory system combinatorial codes and the sensitivity of this process is often underestimated.

Stuart Firestein, Columbia University's Professor of Biological Sciences and a world-renowned olfaction scientist, expressed the wonder of our nose's talents during a hugely successful TED talk aptly titled 'The pursuit of ignorance'. He suggested we take the smell of pears and bananas as an example. For me, a pear's smell is fruitier, fresher and evokes notions of juiciness, while banana is gentle and talc-like or perhaps a little starchy when not ripe, becoming more potent and sickly sweet as the fruit darkens and ripens. At a structural level, pear odour (heptyl acetate) and banana (hexyl acetate) are both made of a chain consisting of a series of carbon, hydrogen and oxygen atoms. The only difference between them is that the pear has an extra carbon atom and two hydrogen ones. And yet our noses clearly identify two distinct and different smells, even if it's difficult to describe them: 'How the hell can we tell the difference between two molecules that differ only by one carbon atom? Surely we are the best chemical detector in the planet and we don't even think about it.'[3]

Modern sensory research and technology such as magnetic resonance imaging (MRI) has revealed exactly which specific regions of the brain light up when a subject sees a face, hears a noise or is touched on the arm. But smell does not need to be constantly connected to the physical source of the stimulus. The smell of your perfume lingers long after you've spritzed your throat and wrists and put the bottle away just as the less pleasant smell of broccoli cooking will haunt the house for hours after you've eaten and washed up.

Ann-Sophie Barwich believes that because the brain processes smell in a very different way from our other senses, it is time to take a different approach to understanding it. Yes, the way we smell is the product of neural activity. But how we perceive the odour in its entirety also depends on what is in our heads in that moment, our past experiences with the scent and how we are feeling in the very moment we smell it. Truly inhaling an odour and really 'feeling' it, she argues, is a layered experience, one coloured by context and personal history, not just the molecular stimulus alone.

A favoured trick of the olfactory boffins to illustrate both chemistry and perception in smell is to blindfold unsuspecting human guinea pigs and ask them to identify two smells, one a lovely chunk of fresh parmesan cheese, the second, freshly produced vomit. The vast majority of subjects will not be able to tell the difference because the major odour molecule, butyric acid, is common to both parmesan and vomit. Once you see what you are smelling (you *know* parmesan, how good it tasted on that pasta, how textured, pungent and crystalline it is on the tongue when fresh) you can rest assured that your perception of the two smells will change dramatically.

A kinder way to conduct a similar exercise requires fruit-flavoured jellybeans, a blindfold and a peg on the nose. Without seeing the colour and the effect of retronasal olfaction releasing odours as you chew, you will not be able to tell the strawberry jellybean from the lemon one or the orange from the vanilla. But as soon as the nose peg is removed, *voilà*, the whole symphony of flavours is back. If the nose peg stays put but you are allowed to see, the likelihood is that you will guess the correct flavour not by smell or taste but by using the sight of its colour as your cue.

If neural activity across the olfactory bulb captures the chemical property of the odour – vomit/parmesan/orange/strawberry – our brain at some point must jettison some information, moving instead to a completely different pattern (dance!) of neural networks, which means that we perceive the odorant in a completely different way from its chemistry. Some of this is affected by culture and what we have grown up to 'know', but so much of the fifth sense remains mysterious and elusive.

2

The Scent of Daffodils

'The flower that smells the sweetest is shy and lowly.' William Wordsworth, one of the great English Romantic poets, wrote these words in 1821. He was a prodigious walker who adored wandering the English countryside composing poetry about the glories of nature – but he could not smell the beauty he observed.

He penned four verses in one afternoon about the joy and beauty of daffodils, their colour and movement – flower heads bobbing and long stems waving as the breeze puffed across the water. But never once did he mention the smell that must have enveloped him as he passed through the golden field, a rich narcissus-like fragrance that can polarise opinion as some perceive it as pleasantly musky or vanilla-ish while others liken it to raw onions, cat urine or even spoiled fish.

A search for the words 'smell', 'scent', 'odour' and 'fragrance' in a six-volume collection of his works published in 1865 and now digitised threw up just half a dozen uses. When he did describe smell, the word he fell back on was 'sweet' – a quality that, even in anosmia, is recognisable by the tongue.

Wordsworth's nephew, the Bishop of Lincoln, Christopher Wordsworth, observed that references to scent in his uncle's poetry were based on what family and friends described to him:

> With regard to fragrance, Mr Wordsworth spoke from the testimony of others: he himself had no sense of smell. The single instance of his enjoying such a perception . . . was, in fact, imaginary. The incident occurred at Racedown [Lodge in Dorset], when he was talking with Miss H [his fiancée Mary Hutchinson], who coming suddenly upon a parterre of sweet flowers, expressed her pleasure at their fragrance, a pleasure which he caught from her lips, and then fancied to be his own.[1]

Wordsworth's friend and fellow poet, Robert Southey, noted twenty years later that once, in youth, the poet's fifth sense had briefly returned:

> Wordsworth has no sense of smell. Once, and only once in his life, the dormant power awakened; it was by a bed of stocks in full bloom, at a house he inhabited in Dorset-shire, some five-and-twenty years ago; and he says it was like a vision of Paradise to him; but it lasted only a few minutes, and the faculty has continued torpid from that time. The fact is remarkable in itself, and would be worthy of notice, even if it did not relate to a man of whom posterity will desire to know all that can be remembered. He has often expressed to me his regret for this privation. I, on the contrary, possess the sense in such acuteness, that

I can remember an odour and call up the ghost of one that
is departed.[2]

The friendship between Southey, passionate and driven by the
sensual pleasures of taste and smell, and Wordsworth, enclosed
in his sensory vacuum, struck me with a profound melancholy.
The notion that Wordsworth was just once able to perceive the
powerful floral scent of stock and lose it again seemed inordinately cruel.

'I am no botanist,' Southey wrote to their friend, the poet and
activist Walter Savage Landor in 1811,

> but, like you, my earliest and deepest recollections are con-
> nected with flowers, and they always carry me back to other
> days. Perhaps this is because they are the only things which
> affect our senses in precisely the same manner as they did in
> childhood. The sweetness of the violet is always the same,
> and when you riffle a rose, and drink, as it were, its fra-
> grance, the refreshment is the same to the old man as to the
> boy. We see with different eyes in proportion as we learn to
> discriminate, and, therefore, this effect is not so certainly
> produced by visual objects. Sounds recall the past in the
> same manner, but do not bring with them individual scenes,
> like the cowslip-field or the bank of violets, or the corner
> of the garden to which we have transplanted field flowers.[3]

Robert Southey's passionate, personal awareness of smell as a
potent mnemonic and pre-eminent sense is intriguing as placing
such value and importance on the sense of smell was a view

unfashionable in his time and few of his contemporaries in the world of the sciences or philosophy agreed with him.

Many of the twenty-first-century cognitive and chemosensory scientists interviewed for this book argue that scientific interest in the fifth sense underwent a relatively recent renaissance that can possibly be dated precisely to April 1991 with reports from Columbia University that two researchers had identified genes in a rat that encoded proteins they predicted were olfactory neurones. This would take some years to prove but it served to ignite an invigorated new interest in understanding a sense that has mystified thinkers from the time of the ancients.

The ancient Greek philosopher Democritus propounded the atomistic theory of smell – an idea that was later picked up by the Roman Lucretius, who concentrated on their 'shape' (remember: round = nice smell atoms; pointy = unpleasant smell atoms). Another of the ancient Greeks, Plato, noted that none of the four elements – earth, air, water and fire – exuded an intrinsic smell, and so proposed an intuitive and prescient theory for smells, which he insisted must surely come from the transformation of the elements into fumes or vapours.

Aristotle took this one step further to suggest that the transmission of odours might require another medium, perhaps air or water, through which odours must pass, envisioning a system of waves that allowed the dissemination of smells and the information they carried. It might appear obvious to us now but Aristotle's theories remain remarkable for his fundamental understanding that one smell from the same source can be perceived completely differently by the individuals smelling it and that reception can depend on state of mind: how hungry you are will affect how you react to the aroma of food cooking, for example.

Thinkers who emerged in later centuries would slowly move away from the predominantly philosophical discussion of smell to a more pragmatic focus, concentrating on the identification and classification of odours and the extraction of substances from aromatic plants, herbs and saps to be used therapeutically.

In medieval times, odours became part of the arsenal of physicians. Most were still guided by the theories of the Greek physician and philosopher Aelius Galenus (129–210), known as Galen of Pergamon, who pioneered clinical observation and reason as essential to diagnosis and prognosis rather than reliance on Roman practices of divination and prophecy. Galen's detailed, clinical observations of the outbreak of a terrible plague that felled millions in 168 CE was so precise that it allowed modern medical historians to identify it as smallpox.[4] He also discovered olfactory organs in the brain and not just in the nose.

The first physician to embrace smell as a diagnostic tool was Ibn Sina widely known in the west as Avicenna (980–1037). He recognised that the odour of urine can change in illness and used his observations in diagnosis – an important tool still used today.

Physicians in the Middle Ages relied on Galen's theories that good health is the result of a fine balance between the 'humours' – bodily fluids including blood, yellow and black biles, and phlegm – as long as they were coupled with their corresponding element. Human bodies, they believed, exude signs of visible and invisible 'humoral' health and odours offered an important clue to the unseen 'balances' within.

How medieval thinkers imagined smells were transmitted continued to follow the reasoning of the ancient Greeks and Romans. They tended towards Aristotle's belief in some form of medium rather than Plato's concept of vapours, often illustrated by the ability of bees to find flowers or vultures cadavers from vast distances even in the absence of wind.

Academic Katelynn Robinson's groundbreaking research into the sense of smell in the Middle Ages reveals in glorious detail the huge significance placed on odour in the texts of both religious and medical scholars of the time, most of which have remained untranslated and unedited in modern academies.[5] Between the thirteenth and fifteenth centuries, medieval scholars translated works from the original Greek or Arabic, often reinterpreting philosophical and medical knowledge and integrating the new beliefs of their own time. Robinson documents how medical authors described the practical application of theories of smell to public health while religious authors reinterpreted knowledge into what she describes as a new 'medically aware theology of smell'.

The fragrances of religious incense, baptismal balms and oils still familiar to us today were inseparable from the rituals of the Church in the Middle Ages. The symbolic importance of smell during this period is demonstrated by a number of objects in the Wellcome Collection – the incredible array of medical antiquities and curiosities amassed by nineteenth-century collector Henry Wellcome. One is a drawing by the sixteenth-century Flemish artist Maerten de Vos, which depicts God breathing life into Adam's nostrils as part of an allegorical representation of the gift of smell.[6]

There was also the belief that saints exuded the fragrance of flowers, while evil, sin and demons brought with them the stench of fire, burning and Hell. This idea that sanctity had its own odour was known as 'osmogenesia' and gave rise to the belief that even the long-dead bodies and relics of Christian saints could produce a sweet and pure floral aroma as a kind of symbolic contrast to the 'sinful' body odours of us mere mortals and sinners.

Changing concepts of personal hygiene and cleanliness also had a profound impact as the Middle Ages drew to a close. Most people lived in unwashed clothing, which was infested with lice, mites and fleas – primary vectors of the plague bacteria. Access to running water and the possibility of heating water for bathing were available only to the very wealthy. The aroma of food cooking, increasingly entwined with fragrant spices brought back from the East after the Crusades, began to be associated with medicinal properties, not just the pleasure of eating. Odours were imbued with powers to purify air indoors and even to prevent disease while bad smells, ubiquitous in growing cities, were seen as portents of fearful diseases such as the plague.

Katelynn Robinson argues that this association of philosophy and medicine reinforced the idea that odours could express evil as well as divinity and, as a result, be seen as the heralds of disease or offer a path to healing. From medieval to Enlightenment Europe, these messages about smell and air were disseminated to the average person from the pulpit via sermons and, later, through laws relating to public health.

The power accorded aromatic herbs and the importance of smell in protecting against 'evil air' and disease is vividly illustrated by the sinister beaked plague masks worn by physicians well into the seventeenth century in Europe. Known widely and still seen in party-costume shops around the world, they were designed to contain protective concoctions of dried flowers, herbs and vinegar-soaked sponges in order to purify the air breathed in by the physician. The mask is said to have been the brainchild of Louis XIII's chief physician, Charles de Lorme, in the mid sixteenth century and its thick leather coverings could well be described as an early equivalent of PPE. A description, translated from the French, noted the

> nose was half a foot long, shaped like a beak, filled with perfume with only two holes one on each side near the nostrils but that can suffice to breathe and carry along with the air one breathes the impression of the herbs enclosed further along in the beak. Under the coat we wear boots made in Moroccan [goat] leather from the front of the breeches in smooth skin that are attached to said boots and a short sleeved blouse in smooth skin, the bottom of which is tucked into the breeches. The hat and gloves are also made of the same skin [and] spectacles over the eyes.[7]

While I was in Naples researching the old perfumer just before the first lockdown, I visited one of the city's best-kept secrets, a perfectly preserved apothecary's pharmacy deep in the heart of the sixteenth-century Hospital for the Incurables and monastic complex. Protected by the impenetrable silence of the Masons for more than three centuries (photographs are still strictly forbidden), it is testament to the place where magic and religion, alchemy, early medicine and the power of early aromatics came into their own.

Inside are more than 500 perfectly preserved ceramic jars decorated with Old Testament scenes but not one of them is labelled with the herbs, powders and fragrant unguents they once contained. Medical historians believe that the early pharmacists learned by heart the contents of the myriad jars by memorising their position and placement on the shelves. As so many were poisonous, this was a form of security against theft or misuse.

Next door to the ancient pharmacy is a small museum where a unique collection of medical instruments is displayed, from amputation tools to a collection of the wooden plague masks – remnants of a time when the fight against terrible, infectious and deadly diseases was believed also to be a war between smells fragrant and foul.

3

From Fragrances Foul

When my sense of smell disappeared so suddenly on that strange afternoon in late March, I was struck most by the sensation of being untethered, as if one of the things that bound me to the world had been wrenched away. In the days that followed, it felt almost as if an internal compass I never knew existed had been excised and the most banal, everyday decisions needed conscious testing by other people. Was the cheese in the fridge still okay? Could anyone else smell smoke?

The olfactory system is constantly on duty for most animals including us humans. Aarhus University's Professor Alexander Fjældstad, a specialist physician and co-founder of Denmark's first outpatient clinic for taste and smell disorders, likens it to a program or app running on your laptop or smartphone. Smells, he says, have a direct shortcut into the part of the brain that relates to 'liking' and pleasurable appreciation but also, importantly, to fear and disgust. 'It is constantly scanning. You don't think about it but your sense of smell is always running there, in the background, and you might not think it's using processing power but it's using quite a lot and all the time.'

The brain doesn't have to work consciously to complete certain types of familiar tasks; it just does them on autopilot. While everything is going to plan, it just whirrs along, quietly scanning and monitoring in the background. But when a spanner is thrown in the works and your brain registers an error, it switches mode to work out what to do next. An experienced driver, for example, changes gear automatically without consciously thinking left foot on clutch, right foot on accelerator, hand on gearstick – familiarity and practice mean your body completes the actions seamlessly and almost unconsciously. However, if someone crosses the road in front of your car without warning, your brain is jolted out of its autopilot mode and immediately signals an alert.

'This is especially so with the sense of smell,' Professor Fjældstad explained, 'because the alert – for example when a [spoiled or toxic] food goes straight into the mouth – it goes directly to the parts of the brain that responds with fear and disgust.'

Sometimes smell works in the opposite way to our other senses. When you see, hear or touch something, the signals are sent to the thalamus, often described as the brain's gateway, which filters information before processing and analysing the stimulus. From there, it is routed to the amygdala, home of emotions and memory. Smell is the only sense that bypasses the thalamus, so when you sniff something, the hit is instant and unconscious – you have a gut reaction first and identification comes shortly after. This is why a toxic food will instantly trigger a gag reflex, instinctive and protective, while a whiff of a familiar cologne can immediately reassure, transporting you instantly back to childhood or a lover's arms.

The idea that our brains and noses are constantly at work, instinctively scanning for touchstones to reassure or alert us made me want to know more about the role of smell and how it was perceived or valued throughout history. We know, for example, that in the late Stone Age, the artists of the Lascaux caves carried lamps made of stone with round cavities to hold animal fats.[1] These would have smoked as they lit the way and combined with the earth and the damp of the walls created a powerful and perhaps evocative scent for the artists who worked inside.

Scholars suggest that for the people of the Magdalenian culture 17,000 years ago, scent already carried an experiential meaning, perhaps protective and even sacred. The word 'perfume' itself is rooted in the Latin which means *per* (by) *fumum* (smoke) and provides verbal illustration of the earliest methods by which the ancients disseminated fragrances, throwing herbs and essences onto a fire. As the perfumed smoke rose to the sky, it was thought to reach the gods, in appeasement or show of gratitude. Contact with such precious essences might have been initially restricted to an elite, priests and healers, great godlike emperors and their courts.

The Egyptians too were masters of fragrance, sending their dead into the afterlife with incenses and scented unguents, cedarwood used in the processes of mummification and to protect against insects. They are the culture credited with discovering techniques of enfleurage – soaking plant material or flower petals in oil before wringing the mixture tightly through cloth to trap and conserve the fragrance. Cleopatra was a legendary connoisseur of the power of perfume and loved bathing in oils of crocus and violet and anointing her hands and feet with lotions of almond oil, honey, cinnamon and orange blossoms. The great ruler and seductress surrounded herself in a cloud of incense and her scent was said to herald her presence even before she could be seen.

Alexander the Great was said to be just as enamoured of the world of fragrance and used both perfumes and incense liberally. The ancient Roman passion for bathing and perfume permeated every aspect of patrician daily life, from petal-soaked pools to the use of perfume on household dogs and horses. There is of course symbolism in the Magi giving scent – frankincense – as a first gift to the baby Jesus, while English lore tells us that a millennium later Edward the Confessor donated what he believed to be an invaluable relic of that first, fragrant gift to Westminster Abbey.

Attitudes to scents and bodily odours have chopped and changed over the centuries, influenced by travel, trade routes east and west and fashions among the elite. In her delicious exploration of the history of the five senses, Diane Ackerman wrote that in the ancient world, even the architecture of potentates was scented, woods chosen for their insect-repellent qualities and the ability to freshen the air. The imperial palace of the Manchu emperors at Ch'eng-te is built of cedarwood while mosques were sometimes fashioned with mortar mixed with rose water and musk and as the sun heated the walls, it would waft perfume over worshippers. 'Ancient he-men were heavily perfumed. In a way, strong scents widened their presence,' she wrote.[2]

In Elizabethan England, body odour was a form of amorous currency. It was common practice for a young woman to peel an apple and place it into her armpit until it absorbed her smell, and then present the fruit to potential suitors as an offering or olfactory aide-memoire of love.[3] In early seventeenth-century France, Louis XIV, who did not like bathing, was reported to have demanded that all the rooms of Versailles be perfumed daily and his clothes washed in aromatic, simmering baths of scented herbs known as 'Acqua Angeli' – water of the angels – essentially a melange of cloves and nutmeg, amber and jasmine. Later in that century, Louis XVI and his wife, Marie Antoinette, employed their own perfumer, Jean-Louis Fargeon, who spent fourteen years in court – until the Revolution cut his career short – concocting ever more sumptuous perfumes for his mercurial client queen.[4]

Napoleon Bonaparte, on the other hand, was a man who famously eschewed artificial scent and during the Italian campaigns of 1796–7 wrote to his lover, Josephine, *'Ne te lave pas, j'accours et dans huit jours je suis là'*, asking that she refrain from bathing so when he returned from battle in eight days, he could enjoy her with all his senses.

This rollercoaster rise and fall in fashions for smells – bodily and artificial – over the centuries is encapsulated by John Trueman, author of *The Romantic Story of Scent*, who wrote: 'The men of the ancient world were clean and scented; the European men of the Dark Ages dirty and unscented; those of Medieval times and up to the seventeenth century dirty and scented and in the nineteenth century, clean and unscented.'

In England, miasma theory – the belief that 'bad air' spread infectious diseases such as cholera and the Black Death – reigned and in the first half of the nineteenth century, as London's population exploded from just over a million people in the census of

1801 to 2.65 million in 1851, it turned the River Thames into one of the most polluted and stinking stretches of water in Europe. Sewage was dumped raw into the river, human and animal refuse piled high and was washed away only by the tidal surges. Flushing toilets, introduced with huge success at the Great Exhibition of 1851, ended up merely adding to the stink as cesspools eventually overflowed, forcing ever more effluent into the river, creeks and canals and backing up into the city at high tides.

The British capital, like its French counterpart, was served by an army of euphemistically named 'night-soil men' (*les boueurs* in France) who collected both liquid and solid human waste, often sold for fertilizer. Conditions were particularly bad in poorer districts of the capital where tanneries and industry produced foul air and death rates were high. In the wealthier suburbs, the residents' better health was attributed to fresher air rather than better living conditions. Throughout most of the nineteenth century, cholera, smallpox and tuberculosis outbreaks were common in European cities.

The need for reform was pressing and physicians and politicians agitating for public-health reform attempted to record in gory detail the effect of the malodorous air on the city's residents. John Hogg, a physician writing in 1837, lambasted the cheek-by-jowl existence of residents with slaughterhouses and burial grounds describing the capital as a 'disgrace', its air 'ever reeking with gore, and steaming with visceral effluvia' and asking why 'burial grounds, fat with human remains, should be tolerated in the midst of a dense population'. Hogg painted a picture of horror as animals, ravaged by exhaustion and thirst, were driven through London's streets and threw themselves onto the torrents of filth in the gutters, often dying 'so the butcher's knife is cheated of its victim'.[5] (He presented a copy of his observations to Queen Victoria in an attempt to push for change and the book remains in the Royal collections.)

Eventually an unusual summer heatwave led to what would become known as the 'Great Stink of 1858', which spurred lawmakers – who of course worked Thames-side in Westminster and the Houses of Parliament – into action, attempting to rid the city of waste through the construction of one of the great engineering feats of the industrialising world – the Victorian sewage system that still flows under London today.

French historian Alain Corbin takes his readers to visit the French capital between the late eighteenth and nineteenth centuries, encouraging us to breathe it in, sniff it, smell it in all its grubby, chaotic, stinking glory. Corbin, who came to the world of smells after an earlier, important body of work and research on the history of prostitution, argued that sometime between the mid eighteenth and late nineteenth century, 'something changes in the way smells are perceived and analysed' by city dwellers.[6]

Corbin recounts a first-hand report of a bitterly cold day in 1782 when a group of Parisian sanitation and public-health experts, including Antoine Lavoisier – often described as the father of modern chemistry – met outside the Hôtel de La Grenade as part of a grand 'public-health' scheme to map the smells of Paris and supervise the emptying and cleaning of its enormous cesspool. The reek is described in stultifying detail, apparently made worse by the dumping of body parts used by medical students into the excrement. Work continues for some hours and chemical substances thrown onto the surrounding snow to mask the fetid air until a workman slips and falls into the mire. He is dragged out unconscious and quickly offered aid by one of the medical experts but the physician suffers a fit inhaling his patient's breath and apparently took many weeks to recover.

For the twenty-first-century reader, the notion that mapping Paris's smells was seen as a life-threatening scientific quest can seem difficult to believe and yet Corbin argues persuasively that over the next century architecture and town planning, medicine, eroticism and gender were all reframed by the shift in societal attitudes to smell. This ultimately led to state-driven, cleansing and street purification campaigns and what he describes as wholesale 'tactics of deodorisation'.[7]

These ranged from engineering triumphs such as underground sewage systems and Baron Haussmann's installation of the 12,000 *bouches de lavage* that still flush Paris's gutters with fresh water today, right through to a kind of 'privatisation' of human ablutions and stink-provoking activities. The deodorisation would also see the end of public latrines and baths, leading to new fashions including the perfuming of homes and domestic spaces – as the aristocracy had done in the past. Smells foul and smells fragrant soon became new indicators of social class and bourgeois refinement. The earliest zoning legislation in many Western cities was essentially a form of segregation of residential areas from industrial areas, spaces delineated by the impact of smell and noise.

The American historian, David S. Barnes, would later focus on the summer months of August and September 1880 in Paris when the city was enveloped in a suffocating cloud of putrid odours, unleashing rumours of unexplained deaths, fury among residents and forcing the formation of an emergency government commission. Scientists were represented on this inquiry body and their report linked the 'pestilential emanations' to the possibility of an epidemic 'any day'.

Fifteen years later, however, when a similar 'great stink' event occurred, germ theory had taken hold so persuasively that the possibility of a smell-induced outbreak of disease was scorned and rejected. According to Barnes, while it was widely accepted by then that smells might be indicative of unhealthy living conditions but were not in themselves a direct danger, high social anxiety about sanitation and bad smells remained: 'No longer life threatening, the odours of Paris remained a threat to a way of life – the civilised, urban life.'[8] A seismic shift had occurred between long-held, scientific and popular ideas about the physical health risks of smell to new ideas about what smells indicated or might signify culturally, about a person's class, education and position in society.

The revolution in civic cleanliness in Western Europe took decades as politicians juggled the demands of employment and energetic resistance from those who earned their living from manual disposal of waste – street sweepers, manure sellers, night-soil men.

As the spectre of infectious diseases such as cholera and typhoid receded and popular acceptance of the new order widened, urban sanitation was soon followed by a similar change in personal hygiene. The earlier belief that it was necessary to leave the skin unwashed to protect it from the malodorous air was replaced by new advice that the skin needed to be cleansed to allow it to release bad fluids and that it needed to 'breathe'.

The cultural historian Constance Classen and her co-authors argue that as the upper and middle classes began to purify their bodies, their homes and their streets of dirt, they grew more conscious of the smells of the working classes. The poor were clearly unable to separate household spaces into bedroom, bathroom, kitchen, dining room in the same way that the wealthy could and odours mingled indiscriminately, 'increasing the revulsion felt towards them by the sensitised bourgeoise, who had come to associate olfactory promiscuity with moral promiscuity'.[9]

A Victorian perfumer, writing in 1891, exemplified even more snobbish attitudes to odours, suggesting that among the 'lower orders' bad smells were simply ignored: 'Noses have they but they smell not. The result is a continuance to live in an atmosphere laden with poisonous odours whereas anyone with the least power of smelling retained shuns such odours as they would anything else that is vile and pernicious.'[10] Morality and smell became intimately linked.

As I read the olfactory histories and adventures, of Alain Corbin, Constance Classen, David Barnes and others, they sparked an odd nostalgia about how much of the world's rich odours we have banished forever from our modern, deodorised world. Nobody would want to return to an age when the streets of our major cities ran with raw sewage, but for me in my bubble of anosmia, well, even the pong of an old drain would have been a welcome relief.

4

Scent and Sensibility

The British chemist Sir William Harry Perkin was already both famous and wealthy in 1868 when, aged just thirty, he wrote an article ponderously titled 'On the Artificial Production of Coumarin and Formation of its Homologues' for the Journal of the Chemical Society of London.[1]

This was a eureka moment for the olfactory world, viewed by perfume historians and smell and flavour scientists as a kind of birthday for modern fragrance chemistry. Perkin's ten-page, formula-thick report for the society described the process he undertook to create synthetic coumarin, an intense, flavourful vanilla-like fragrant which in nature comes from the strange and wrinkly tonka bean, aromatic seed of a huge tree that lives deep in the Amazon forests. The contemporary biophysicist and perfume historian Luca Turin describes the tonka bean as having a 'wonderful, sweet, nutty herbaceous tobacco-like smell'[2] while chefs familiar with the ingredient report that when grated in tiny amounts into desserts or infused into sweet syrups, it imparts a flavour so transcendent that it was dubbed by the BBC the 'most delicious ingredient you've never heard of'.[3] (Tonka bean eaten in larger amounts can also be poisonous.)

Ancient alchemists and perfumers had spent millennia learning to extract, mix, heat, mince and trap fragrance from organic materials, efforts given a huge technological fillip in Italy in the fourteenth century when a new type of distillery cooling system was developed that paved the way for the production of high-grade, pure and clear alcohol. Subsequently, this meant ingredients could be separated from each other, diluted and mixed in varying concentrations, allowing creative experimentation to see how odorants smelled on the skin or changed as they evaporated over varying periods of time.

Sir William Perkin had made his first important discovery when he was barely eighteen years old. He had been tinkering in a makeshift lab in the family home during the Easter holidays, obsessed with trying to synthesise quinine for the treatment of malaria when he found himself with a beaker full of a luminous, deep-purple-coloured liquid. (The word malaria itself is a hangover of the miasma theories of the past: the Latin *mal aria* means 'bad air'.) Serendipity had led the young chemist to create the first synthetic fabric dye, 'mauveine', a find that would later lead to the creation of a torrent of vivid and richly hued dyes, revolutionising the way textiles were coloured and making Perkin a very rich and famous man.

Coumarin would be just as significant and lead to as many significant ramifications for scent: it could mimic the ephemeral, rare and extremely expensive tonka bean but for a fraction of the price. Perkin's synthetic coumarin, often described in perfume literature as the smell of 'new mown hay or grass' would spark the race for other, man-made formulas not just for the perennially fashionable floral scents such as rose, violet and bergamot but for the most rare and prestigious, status-marking perfuming ingredients such as sweet-smelling ambergris, which develops inside the intestine of sperm whales and is excreted in great, grey waxy lumps into the sea to be found washed up on shorelines primarily around the Atlantic ocean.

Ambergris is one of the most intriguing of odorants, in the past called 'floating gold' or 'treasure of the sea' and used for millennia. It smells faecal when first expelled by the whale but over months and years of saltwater and sunshine, develops a hardened texture imbued with a peculiar odour described at once as sweet, earthy, marine and animal-ish. Herman Melville in *Moby Dick* described the terrible odour exuded by a long-dead whale but from which 'stole a faint stream of perfume' and observed a great irony in that 'fine ladies and gentlemen should regale themselves with an essence found in the inglorious bowels of a sick whale'.[4]

By the 1870s, chemists had cottoned on to the fact that if cooked up cheaply in the laboratory, compounds that mimicked such scarce and evocative fragrances could be significant money-spinners. Soon after, a man-made heliotropin was fashioned, a gentle fragrance reminiscent of both vanilla and mimosa flowers. Vanillin would follow, synthesised from pinewood sap in the laboratory by German chemists but until then extracted at great cost from fermenting vanilla pods. A duo of Czech-Austrian scientists were next to crack the formula for quinolines, tongue-curling bitter smells that in tiny amounts imparted a pleasurable leathery tone, and in 1888 the most striking of all, the discovery of nitro-musks by the German chemist Albert Baur.

Like ambergris, musk was immensely expensive and difficult to source, scraped cruelly from the sex glands of the male Asian musk deer. In its concentrated form, it is apparently unpleasant but has been used since antiquity as a scent perceived as intrinsically carnal, both seductive and mysterious. Heaven knows who thought to harass the poor musk deer to source it first. Like Perkin's, Baur's find was accidental: he had been working on the explosive trinitrotoluene (TNT), trying to tweak its molecular structure in an effort to get more bang for productive buck, when he added what are known as the tert-butyl group of chemicals only to unleash an unusual and pleasurable smell in his laboratory – one that reminded him immediately of musk.

Baur knew this was a valuable and potentially prestigious ingredient not just for its scent but also because it was used to slow down evaporation of perfumes' ingredients, a kind of natural fixative that also improved the tenacity of perfume aromas. He quickly patented his 'Musk Baur' and many others would follow, including musk ambrette and musk ketone – all aroma chemicals that ensured that he too became a very rich chemist. And so, dyes, inks, artificial scents and tastes – all became intertwined as the nascent fragrance and flavour chemistry industries began to blossom and grow.

In the centuries between the end of the Dark Ages and the Industrial Revolution that sparked the boom in perfume production, philosophers were also tussling with questions about man's role in nature. During the Renaissance, theologians used biblical texts to show that animals were placed on Earth solely for man's use. As Genesis 11:2 decreed: 'And the fear of you and the dread of you shall be upon every beast of the earth, and upon every fowl of the air, upon all that moveth upon the earth, and upon all the fishes of the sea; into your hand are they delivered. Every moving thing that liveth shall be meat for you; even as the green herb have I given you all things.'[5] Classical moralists countered with a return to the thought of the ancients, among them Plato's reminder (via Socrates) that in every man lies something of the 'lawless, wild beast nature' capable of any notion of 'folly or crime' given the right circumstance.[6]

The lives of animals, with their earthy and indecorous habits – including an olfactory interest in the bodies of their fellow creatures – were something to be scorned, observed the Scottish-born Australian evolutionary zoologist D. Michael Stoddart, and it was the job of religion and morality to curb these undesirable traits and haul man 'above the brute creation'.

'Man was unique; a creature of God's will, which was set far apart from the beasts of the field whose outward signs of civility, decorum and politeness were so marked that René Descartes developed his famous doctrine that animals were mere machines while man alone combined matter and intellect,' Professor Stoddart wrote in his seminal book *The Scented Ape.*[7] A century after Descartes published his *Meditations*, arguing that the human senses alone cannot be trusted when man is trying to determine the nature of reality, his compatriot epistemologist Étienne Bonnot de Condillac proposed an imaginary exercise in which a 'man-statue', empty of any pre-conceived ideas or sense-impressions, is granted the five senses, one by one, in order to examine the process of knowledge acquisition.[8] De Condillac began his treatise with the fifth sense because in his mind, smell contributes least to the human intellect.

The German philosopher, Immanuel Kant, would also dismiss smell, describing it as 'the most dispensable' of the senses:

> Which organic sense is the most ungrateful and also seems the most dispensable? The sense of smell. It does not pay to cultivate it or to refine it at all in order to enjoy; for there are more disgusting objects than pleasant ones (especially in crowded spaces) and even when we come across something fragrant, the pleasure coming from the sense of smell is fleeting and transient.[9]

The idea that man's illustrious image might be compared with those of the animals over which he had been sent to reign would dominate philosophical thought for two centuries. But then, noted Professor Stoddart with palpable glee, 'along came Charles Darwin'. Publication of the Victorian naturalist's groundbreaking *On the Origin of Species* on 24 November 1859, suggesting that man had descended from the apes – the very same wild animals gaped at by thousands of visitors to Britain's Victorian zoos – was greeted by a theological and moralistic storm. His pioneering work would later be seen as the launch of a new scientific discipline, evolutionary biology, and yet even Darwin, in his *Descent of Man*, published twelve years later, would join the philosophers and scientific men of the past to dismiss the olfactory sense as being of 'extremely slight service, if any, even to the dark-coloured races of men, in whom it is more highly developed than in the white and civilised races'.[10]

Perhaps thinkers and scientists of the eighteenth and nine-teenth century found it particularly difficult to grapple with smell because it was altogether too transient, intangible and unmeasurable to take seriously in humans – particularly in comparison with other senses such as vision and touch.

Two decades later, the French neuroanatomist and anthropologist Paul Broca further cemented notions that smell was the poor cousin of the other senses. Broca had observed that humans had larger frontal lobes than those of other animals and that we possess language and complex cognitive capacities that other animals do not. However, because human olfactory bulbs are smaller than those seen in other animals and we don't display the kind of overt sniffing and smelling behaviours of many of our fellow mammals, Broca extrapolated that evolutionary and adaptive changes had shrunk our olfactory capacities.

He then listed animals into two groups – as 'osmatic' or 'anosmatic' – depending on the size of the olfactory lobe. While he accepted that humans remained sensitive to smell, he threw us into the basket with primates and marine mammals such as whales based on the argument that our olfactory powers were 'considerably lessened'. Broca did not embark on sensory research or specific studies to prove his theory but the notion that we rely more on thought than primal senses for survival stuck.[11] John P. McGann, a neuroscientist at Rutgers University, argues that scientists over the years simply built new layers onto this shaky foundation.[12]

As sense of smell was being dismissed, vision was being championed. Half a century later, Sigmund Freud argued that human beings pass through a mini-process of evolution, growing from dependent, prone infants into quadrupeds and on to independence, walking upright. During growth, infantile acuity of smell and pleasure in maternal odours is high but should give way to the 'higher', mature pleasures offered by vision as they grow. Individuals who continue to focus on the olfactory exhibited a form of arrested psychological development.

I love the less Freudian and more medically straightforward theory propounded by the American psychologist and chemosensory scientist Dr Avery Gilbert. In his book *What the Nose Knows* (a constant companion to me throughout my anosmia), Gilbert argues that Freud's regular bouts of sinusitis, nose surgery, cocaine use, cigar smoke and, finally, ageing, left him with a clinically impaired sense of smell – hyposmia. 'Freud's nose was already a disaster zone when he hatched his smell theory in 1897 and my hunch is that he was already smell impaired.'[13]

Not everyone subscribed to the idea of smell being a useless sense. Havelock Ellis, the delightfully named English physician who challenged Victorian taboos about discussion of human sexuality, described it as an exceedingly sensitive if often neglected sense. He saw it as important to human sexuality, suggesting that bodily odours communicate both identity and familiarity. However, he too put another nail in the coffin of the fifth sense by linking it with various abnormal 'nervous conditions' and warning that some odours could themselves spark a particular type of 'neurasthenia'. Some professions, Havelock Ellis added, were also particularly vulnerable to this kind of dementia, among them those that dealt in scent such as 'musk dealers' and even poets and novelists who described olfactory experiences in their writing.[14]

As the twentieth century rolled on, more resources and research effort were ploughed into understanding the physiology and science of sight – seen as an imperative for education and employment – and a more vision-centric view of the world began to dominate. As a result, the significance of smell appeared to decline even further. Mark Jenner, Professor of Early Modern History at the University of York, cites several thinkers, among them Norbert Elias,[15] the German sociologist and author of *The Civilising Process* in the early 1930s, and, a decade later, the French historian Lucien Febvre, who believed that man's propensity towards smell faded as social norms and societal structures became more complex. The fact that sight and hearing were deemed necessary to the efficient functioning of a working adult in the modern world 'helped deaden smell in favour of sight', wrote the American sensory historian, Mark Smith.[16]

✻

D. Michael Stoddart, a biologist, zoologist and now professor emeritus at the University of Tasmania, published his seminal *The Scented Ape* in 1990. His examination of the shift in the significance of odours in human life was among the first to question the role of smell through the lens of evolutionary biology and to ask if Western societies' loss of interest in bodily smells and the natural odours of reproduction might be as much the result of evolutionary adaptation as cultural change. Stoddart noted that we humans possess more scent-secreting areas over our bodies than any of the other primates – hence the title of his book. In the West we have become so punctilious about stripping ourselves of any form of body odour that perhaps he should have called his book *The Sanitised Ape*.

Nearly two decades after this work, Professor Stoddart turned his attention to try to explain, once again through the lens of adaptive biology, why it might be that we've spent two millennia trying to change our bodily smells when no such behaviour is seen in other mammals. Stoddart uses the discovery of a genetic mutation that occurred in our primate ancestors around 16 million years ago to offer a theory to explain our unusual olfactory habits. The University of Michigan biologists who identified the genetic mutation believe it occurred around 23 million years ago, just before what are known as Old World monkeys and hominids separated.[17] In effect, the specific set of genes and smell receptors that encoded pheromones were deactivated, ending the passage of information between the vomeronasal organ (or VNO), which is in the mouth (above the palate in other primates), and the brain. This effectively meant that all those millions of years ago, the earliest humans could no longer 'smell' female ovulation, the main driver of the reproductive habits of primates and many other terrestrial vertebrates.

For us humans at least, smell was no longer the main, powerful and dominant force governing sexual activity – and despite what the perfume industry might tell us, we are not behaviourally driven by 'pheromones'. In his most recent work, *Adam's Nose and the Making of Humankind*, Professor Stoddart goes further to argue that this important evolutionary change might also explain humans' unique (serial) monogamy, arguing it stymied the need for violent, often life-threatening competition for fertile females and ensured that human offspring, dependent and vulnerable for much longer than their animal counterparts, were more likely to be given longer care by their parents.[18] While this part of his argument has been greeted with spirited opposition from some anthropologists who are not swayed by a predominantly biological explanation for human mating habits, the possibility that bodily smells play a minor part in human attraction makes the ongoing, ancient passion for new scents even more intriguing.

The stories of Sir William Perkin, Albert Baur and many other pioneers of synthetic chemistry show that the drive to find man-made compounds to mimic natural fragrances accelerated because the market for new odours to mask or perhaps silently complement bodily smells continued to flourish. Chemistry meant that producers could bypass the unpredictability and seasonal limits of flower harvests, a staple of perfumes and scent manufacture for millennia, as well as offering alternatives for odorants that came from animals that were not just rare and punishingly expensive but also starting to raise ethical and environmental dilemmas.

By the twentieth century, observed Ann-Sophie Barwich, the difference between a natural scent, crafted from natural ingredients, and a fragrance created in a laboratory five minutes ago, became strangely uncertain raising intriguing new questions about what it means to 'perceive' a smell over what constitutes the odour itself.

5

Beauty without Smell

While thinkers, ancient and modern, have wrestled with the complexity and mysteries of our fifth sense, there is one twenty-first-century philosopher who has spent decades asking herself what it means to perceive the world without an olfactory dimension. Marta Tafalla is Associate Professor of Philosophy at the Universitat Autònoma in Barcelona. Born without a sense of smell, a condition known as congenital anosmia, Tafalla became fascinated with her own subjective perception of the world, one she says she found increasingly difficult to explain even as time passed.

Congenital anosmia, she observes, means she has no experience of perfumes and pleasurable fragrances but also no understanding of the stenches that can trigger disgust. For her, smells simply do not exist. But equally, because she has never had these sensations, she makes clear that she does not perceive the world as incomplete. When she sees a cherry tree in full bloom, she gazes at its branches rising upward to the sky, observes it is laden with flowers, hears the wind blow through its leaves and absorbs the whiteness of the flowers in contrast with the vibrant red of the fruit.

Hers is an aesthetic pleasure untrammelled by the feeling that something is missing or that there is a hidden part of the tree – its scent – that escapes her. The notion that others can perceive another dimension of reality, one that requires inhalation of chemical particles 'read' by the mere act of breathing feels as alien to her as the eco-location system used by bats or the abstract understanding that some birds have the capacity to align their flight with the earth's magnetic field.

As an exercise to try to explain this, Tafalla asks those who can smell to imagine walking with her into a fictional world where a small group of hereditary anosmics emigrate together to an island and build their own society, one where nobody has a sense of smell. Over generations, their language would broaden as the culture grew but it would have no words related to smell. The anosmics would prepare and cook food but probably choose to eat in a very different way, driven primarily by colour and texture over the nuance of flavour. Repulsive stenches wouldn't be a problem, skunks ignored, kids wouldn't make stink bombs or laugh at farts.

The settlers' descendants wouldn't even be aware of the existence of another dimension – until a traveller arrives in their world to tell them of the myriad wonderful sensations that they're missing. 'The only thing that can free us anosmics from our island is the words of other people. What makes me aware that my perception of reality is incomplete is that other people talk about sensations that I cannot share. Their stories reveal to me that I lack something,' she told me.

Estimates vary but clinicians generally agree that congenital anosmia occurs in around one in 10,000 births. Typically, children are not diagnosed until their teens when they themselves become aware that they are missing something their peers are sharing. Parents often report feeling guilty that they did not notice sooner or will look back on a particular incident in childhood which suddenly takes on meaning. Tafalla recalls that neither she nor her family was aware that she was born without a sense of smell and despite childhood visits to the doctor for routine tests, olfaction was never checked. As a child, she didn't have the feeling of something missing, although she remembers feeling confusion when her father would talk about the smell of dinner cooking or when she was told to put out the garbage because it stank. 'I saw people breathe in and I did the same, but it brought nothing interesting. Was there something wrong with the way I breathed?'

As a young person, there was a sensation of discomfort only when this absence was pointed out by other people's words but understanding that her perception of the world was different from that of other people would have required an exercise in sophisticated abstraction that is very difficult for a child. It would be a series of small incidents, including being in trouble with a sports teacher at boarding school for not washing her stinky feet, that finally led to the understanding that she could not smell. However, it took a couple more years to find the courage to utter the words 'I cannot smell' to her parents.

Later, a visit to the paediatrician with her concerned mother led to the dismissive diagnosis that 'it's not important', which served to alleviate her mother's anxiety. 'Over the following years I posed the same question to different doctors but only to receive the same answer. Unfortunately, in those years – all this was happening in the 1980s – I never met a single doctor or anybody else who considered that olfaction played a key role in health.'

Tafalla observes that telling people she cannot smell often elicits exactly the same response, although she has classified the most common reactions to her anosmia into four different 'types'. There are those like the doctor who dismiss it as unimportant; those who exclaim she should feel fortunate because she can't smell bad things; those who acknowledge and want to engage and talk about the complexity of explaining smell (her favourite type); and those who listen to her story but then five minutes later ask her to smell their new perfume, making her feel they simply weren't listening. 'This has been the most frequent response. It has happened to me all my life, with my family, my friends, with academics, with scientists interested in olfaction and even several times with my mother,' she wrote. 'Because it is so generalised, I can understand that there is no bad intention, but I see that anosmia just does not mean anything to these people. They don't realise what it means not to be able to smell.'

Tafalla pretty much ignored her lack of smell for many years, having made the decision to live happily in her world without olfactory dimension, spending long periods without even remembering that odours existed. Then, at the age of thirty-four, she had an experience that would change her life. It was 2006 and she was in London in springtime. Away from family and friends, she was free to spend her days and nights working on a postgraduate research project examining the aesthetic appreciation of natural landscapes, immersed in reading about perception. While she was reading about deafness, she was struck by the realisation that the lack of a sense really does change your relationship with the world. In an instant, she became focused on the fifth sense and her own anosmia, feverishly linking ideas, remembering experiences, reflecting on anecdotes and earlier discussions about smell. She stopped her research work and began to write about anosmia, at last finding a way to acknowledge and think about it and for the first time, talking and sharing the experience with others.

Inspired, she then decided she should write a novel, a fictional tale of a child who, after being diagnosed with anosmia, sets out to travel the world in search of a cure. The little child read from *Tales from the Arabian Nights* and became obsessed and immersed in the city of Baghdad, swirling with the smells of spice and perfumes, and became convinced it was there she would find her cure. Tafalla says writing the book was a little like sitting on a therapist's couch, a form of self-psychoanalysis. But it also seeded a fierce intellectual curiosity to explore and understand the physiology of olfaction, the perception of smells and its relationship with the other senses.

The following year, while attending a summer school on landscape and art, she met Teresa Garcerán, a garden designer who had lost her sense of smell the year before. This was the first time she had met someone who had experienced both worlds: 'Teresa was very generous and patient with me . . . she was the first person to tell me that when one loses olfaction, the world changes in a radical way. After that I read that some people who lose their sense of smell go through a period of sadness, frustration or even depression,' she recalled. 'I began to think that between the anosmic world and one containing smells, there must be an abyss.'

Her novel *Nunca sabrás a qué huele Bagdad* (*You Will Never Know How Baghdad Smells*) was published in 2010 and this too propelled her headlong into a new phase of learning and exploration that saw her meet many more people interested in olfaction, from otolaryngologists to philosophers to marketing specialists to chemosensory scientists as well as many more people with anosmia, both acquired and congenital.

Collecting and analysing conversations with this group led to her being able to write and explain in detail what information anosmics are missing out on in day-to-day life and, conversely, to help shine some light on the anosmic experience for those who can smell: 'Thanks to talking with them, I have come to understand that I am missing information about what goes on around me and that I am missing emotional experiences,' she says. Her earliest research work, entitled 'A World without the Olfactory Dimension', has also branched out to explore anosmics' aesthetic appreciation.[1] I felt as if she had opened a new world to me as I read her observations about several remarkable aspects of anosmic perception, words that eloquently expressed some ephemeral and yet profound aspects of 'being' I had never considered.

For example, Tafalla argues that the horizon is experienced very differently by anosmics because it stops at the limit of vision. Those who can smell can often perceive things that lie well beyond sight. In the city, you might know there's a baker around the corner before you see it or know the cafe is open and making espressos or that there is a shop selling bath products nearby. Walking in forests and woodlands, people with normal olfactory function can sense the sea is close even if it is out of sight or that nearby fields have been strewn with manure or recently mown.

While these odours provide less precise information than that offered by sight, they help with a sense of orientation and, Tafalla says, are probably particularly significant at night. 'Odour generates a sense of surrounding, it has something like an enveloping effect . . . I thought that smells were more finite, more like smoke columns. Now I realise that they fill the space where they are and envelop the people who are there, perhaps in a way that is similar to how light fills a space.'

For anosmic people, places feel more empty, whereas sight and hearing reinforces the sensation of distance. For example, those without a sense of smell have no perception of a stuffy room, or if spaces such as restaurants or railway carriages are too crowded to feel comfortable. 'I think that when I perceive my surroundings, my sensation will always be that they are more empty,' she observes.

For those who can smell, people and places also have distinctive odours, olfactory characteristics that help us create an emotional map because they might have been associated with pleasure, evoking familiarity, emotion or simply because they offered a unique, fragrant experience. Of course, the opposite is also true and we can remember places and, sadly, people too for their gut-wrenching stench. Tafalla's observation that the loss of smell during adulthood can also destroy some internal, emotional maps resonated with me: when you lose olfaction you lose a key piece of information about a place as well as your emotional connection with it. For anosmics who have never been handed this part of the emotional jigsaw, it simply does not arise.

Similarly, time can take on different characteristics when the anosmic experience is compared to that of a person who can smell. The intensity of memory evoked by smell has undoubtedly been experienced by all those who have the fifth sense, inspiring writers and poets, most famously Marcel Proust, who described it as 'involuntary memory' in his now oft-(over)-quoted transportation back to childhood as he dipped a delicate madeleine into a cup of tea.[2]

On the other hand, olfaction also represents a kind of anticipatory force because those of us who can smell can know something is going to happen or it can reveal things still hidden to sight. Tafalla tells of a young journalist she met who knew as soon as she stepped into the lift in her apartment block if her father had already returned home, so distinct but also familiar was his scent to her. Smell can provoke a sense of anticipation of what is to come. 'I believe that this anticipatory function is what inspires the metaphorical use of olfaction as a form of intuition,' observes Tafalla. When it is said that someone has a good sense of smell, it can suggest that they have a good sense of things that are not visible or are perhaps hidden and, she notes, is often used metaphorically in detective novels or films. Anosmics don't see what is no longer there or what has yet to come, perceiving only the present: 'I think that anosmic people live more in the present than people with olfaction.'

Philosophers, argues Tafalla, have also grappled with notions of aesthetic appreciation for millennia and yet from Plato to the thinkers of the mid twentieth century most have insisted that aesthetic appreciation is dominated by sight and hearing. When a garden is perceived, it is absorbed by all the senses but often, when the time comes to utter a judgement about it, only sight – 'that garden is beautiful' – is the sense used.[3]

Historically, smell has been placed on the lower rungs of the hierarchy of the senses, regarded as less reliable, more primitive in its connection with bodily or biological responses. When we contemplate the cherry tree in an aesthetic way alone – not for its capacity to produce delicious fruit – it is devoid of any practical utility and therefore unconnected to any biological need. 'Aesthetics is pleasure of the mind, not of the body: we can even say that it is an ascetic pleasure,' says Tafalla. 'And philosophers thought that only sight and hearing allow this rise from the biological to the cognitive level because olfaction, taste and touch are too closely tied to biological needs; to hunger, thirst, fear, sexual desire – in short to the body.'

As a philosopher herself, she felt moved to join fellow academics, including Professor Barry Smith, his American colleague Professor Carolyn Korsmeyer, and Manchester University's Professor Jim Drobnick, who have all questioned these notions and written about aesthetic appreciation as a product of all our senses working separately and together. But Tafalla wanted to examine and compare the lack of olfaction in the aesthetic value of things: 'When we anosmic people look at a garden or a forest without noticing a smell, do we find them more beautiful or more ugly? What are the differences in aesthetic appreciation with and without smell?'[4]

I found her conclusions intriguing and unexpected: she argues that for the anosmic the world is not quite as beautiful as that of the person who can smell but that at the same time it is also less ugly. She cites the example of a big public park near where she lives in Barcelona that is planted with lots of aromatic but visually rather uninteresting Mediterranean plants. To those that can smell them, the herbaceous borders have a particular and powerful aesthetic value but to those who cannot, they're almost boring, lacking elegant shapes, distinctive foliage or flowers. This feeling that she might be missing something others enjoy very much bothered her so much that she decided to plant some in pots on her patio as a way of providing pleasure for others – with the exception of the young daughter of a friend, the only one to find the smells overpowering and unpleasant. The value that her visitors place on the aromas of the plants suggests that if she could smell, there would indeed be some things that would seem more beautiful to her. 'I could say the same thing about many natural settings, and also about food, tea and wine.'

Perhaps one of the strangest aspects of smell loss lies in the vacuum where other people's smells are – and where our own body odour is. For me, the experience of anosmia meant I no longer could smell myself and it felt as if I'd somehow disappeared, my sense of self stripped of a layer, triggering niggling anxiety about what others might be perceiving. Being born without a sense of smell means Tafalla has simply never experienced this aspect of herself. She acknowledges too that her relationship with other people at a cognitive level must surely be missing a layer, one that tells others but not her that they share an office with a colleague infamous for not showering after the gym or to understand a friend's ability to be able to discern if her two daughters have switched clothes or slept in each other's beds. 'I have access to this information only if someone else shares it with me, in which case I have to trust their word. Perhaps all this means that I don't know people as well as others do,' she says. 'Popular culture says love is blind. In my case it is blind and anosmic. I do not know whether this is unfortunate or, on the contrary, good luck!'

In Umeå, northern Sweden, where Lars Lundqvist lives with his wife, horses, cats and a working cocker spaniel, it is a midsummer evening. While the sun has set in London, his home – at 64°N – is roughly the same latitude as Fairbanks in Alaska and still flooded with daylight. As an Associate Professor with the Faculty of Forest Sciences in Umeå, Lundqvist's professional and research path is dominated by the life of trees, specifically the biomechanics of their growth in forests of uneven age. But I have not asked to talk to him about silviculture. I am intrigued by his book, *A World Without Smells*.[5]

Like Marta Tafalla, Dr Lundqvist was born congenitally anosmic, and I am keen to hear what it is like to work inside nature but to be unable to smell it or even imagine its odours. Lundqvist had read Tafalla's work but had more questions to ask. Why is it that we would not expect a congenitally blind person to understand colour or to distinguish between day and night but congenital anosmics – if noticed at all – are often treated as if they're not trying hard enough to share the perceptions of those around them? Early on in our chat, Lundqvist makes clear that he does not like the description 'nose blind':

If you're deaf, you wouldn't want to be called 'ear blind'. It is a pity there isn't a more common word – anosmia is a tricky word not familiar like blind or deaf. Also, there seems to be a difference in how it is used: people say 'I'm blind' or 'I am deaf' and yet in Sweden at least, they say 'I have anosmia' – but for me, for us in the group, we say 'we are anosmic', it is not an illness it is the way we are.

Lundqvist's own book on anosmia is relatively short, unadorned and yet profound in its unsentimental explanation of life without smell. It was an eye opener for me as an acquired (and temporary) anosmic and I wondered what had finally pushed him to examine his own experience. His observations are matter of fact, untrammelled by the profound sense of mourning and loss that forms so much of the experience of those who lose their fifth sense through illness or trauma.

We often discuss this on the Facebook group for congenital anosmics because some people even get annoyed by seeing how upset others are when they have lost it. But to us, it's 'who cares' it is not that important! It's a very strange and difficult point of view to explain it or to understand it . . .

I think it is the same for most people who are congenitally blind, deaf or anosmic when we are alone, we don't think much about it, it just is.

The air he breathes, he says, is the same inside his home or outside in the woodlands. It is the same whether he's mucking out the horses' stables or plugging a leaking sewerage pipe while his family gag, incredulous around him. There is no difference between the air that enters his nose while he is walking through a field of wildflowers or sitting by his sick child's bed with the vomit bucket beside it. 'This is the biggest difference with people who can smell,' he tells me. 'The environment always changes, depending on smell. My environment is only what I can see and what I can hear so the air is exactly the same everywhere.'

His work in forestry and obvious appreciation and love of nature made me immediately think about William Wordsworth who would have lived in a similar universe, moved profoundly to write poetry about the natural environment that surrounded him, aware of others' olfactory responses and yet experiencing it solely through sight and hearing.

Speaking in the easy, elegant English of those educated in Scandinavia, Lundqvist ascribes the decision to write about living without smell to 'what was probably some kind of revelation': 'It dawned on me not just that *I* was missing this whole concept and didn't understand smell but also realising that nobody else understood it either. This was really shocking.'

While many acquired anosmics are immediately driven to search for information about their condition, he felt the desire to explore a new understanding only in his mid fifties, turning first to Swedish health authorities, who, surprisingly, referred him to disability organisations who in turn referred him back to health departments. This would be the first lesson learned – that the wider medical world seemed to know as little about his condition as he did.

Knowing that olfaction bypasses the thalamus for immediate processing by the amygdala and that this instinctive, primitive response is often protective, I'm curious to know if anything does disgust him. 'No, it doesn't. Someone who knows how faeces and vomit smells associates the sight of such things with feelings of disgust. So, just seeing something like that without smelling it can cause nausea but not to me,' he says. 'I guess that is the upside . . . when the kids were sick and vomiting I could sit with them, clean it up. It doesn't bother me.' For me, even hearing somebody talk about vomit can occasionally trigger a gag reflex while discussion about fetid smells or events over dinner can ruin your appetite. But having never made that connection at all – and these are learned responses as children often will play with their own faeces before they're taught not to – Lundqvist says he simply doesn't recognise this feeling, writing a chapter titled 'Nothing is Disgusting' to try to explain it.

As a child, he taught himself to respond 'correctly' in a normosmic world by watching and mimicking others. I wonder out loud if he thinks this is the same process that children on the autistic spectrum undergo to learn to respond socially or to facial expressions and he nods in agreement. Often, he was driven by the natural desire to fit in with his peers, laughing at farts or smell jokes. Later, it would be to avoid having to explain that he had no response to everyday observations such as 'Doesn't the bacon smell good?' or 'We're getting close to the coast. Can you smell the sea?' Reading this part of his experience, I felt viscerally how tiring it must be to try to behave in a way that is not instinc-tive. Years later, as a young teenager, it often just became easier to copy the answers others gave and nod in assent. In retrospect, this constant need to conform added layers of existential stress that he had failed to acknowledge for decades until he decided to write about his experience.

His way of managing was to establish rules to cover these aspects of day-to-day life and, as long as he abides by them, he feels safe in the knowledge he is not provoking anyone or 'behaving like a misfit'. But even a passing comment about smells such as 'What's that smell? Where is it coming from?' can still provoke anxiety. 'I can understand intellectually that it is a rhetorical question – but such questions always feel unfair and subconsciously they feel like criticism, accusing me of being too dumb to understand smells. But how could I? Could a congenitally blind person know that a light bulb needs changing?' As we spoke, it didn't surprise me to read that his anosmia had also resulted in a store of anger and frustration, another catalyst to want to write about it.

At the same time, Lundqvist insists he has no desire to be someone else and while he is aware that so much of the world – from cooking programmes on television to the enjoyment of nature – is reliant on smell, anosmia also defines who he feels he is. Sharing what his family and friends know and experience every day would be a wonderful thing, he adds, but this isn't what affects him most. 'What probably hurts is this despair of never really being understood by people around me. That they never really understand that I do not know what smells are and no matter how hard I try to memorise the rules and try to behave correctly, I simply do not know what they're talking about!'

●

Chatting with Lundqvist that late summer evening, I realised I'd been assuming that those born with anosmia would be more comfortable and accustomed to navigating the world without their fifth sense than those who had developed the condition. And yet Lundqvist is forthright about the integral role played by his wife in his quest to learn how to manage the activities that punctuate the most banal rhythms of day-to-day life. Shared jobs such as cleaning the house are rarely smooth sailing for any of us. He describes his wife as a super nose, always aware of the joyous scent of nature, flowers and woodlands but equally sensitive and ready to comment about food past its best, damp towels, used shirts, garbage. Issues of hygiene and cleanliness became a source of repeated familial tension: 'I never thought I would react to those kind of comments but, wow, suddenly I realised that I did. My world is essentially clean,' he smiles. 'I started to think about the book in what was like a crisis moment, because I had not realised how much it affected me but also my relationship.'

These days, there is much more discussion about the sensory abyss between them, even laughter at times. Not long ago, he recalls, she asked if he would like her to bake cinnamon or cardamom buns. When he told her it made no difference, she looked at him 'like it was the most stupid thing to say'. 'Until then, I thought cinnamon or cardamom was the shape of the bun, not what you put in it. I had honestly never made the connection,' he laughed. 'And I can tell the difference now because the cardamom bun contains more butter and is stickier.' His wife has since stopped asking about cooking ingredients such as spices or if he would like fresh herbs in a stew and now simply points out when a towel or shirt needs changing without comment: 'In a way it would have been nice to have the book forty years ago. It would have helped in some situations,' he adds, almost as an afterthought.

However, for me it is his explanation of the more philosophical, unique aspects of his existence, expressed by comparing his own experience with his wife's, that I found most illuminating.

He says he was both inspired and informed by Tafalla's writing. 'When my wife and I walk in a forest, we see trees, plants, rocks and we hear birds, possibly insects, the wind and so on,' he wrote. 'But on top of that my wife will also be surrounded by the smells of the forest. The smells will amplify the sensation of being in exactly that kind of forest and will thereby also amplify the perception of the surrounding space. If she closes her eyes, she can still sense the forest around her. When I close my eyes, the sounds remain and nothing else. In a way, the forest disappears when it is no longer visible.' Tafalla, he says, also made him think deeply about the relationship between smells and the spaces that surround us and the understanding that they can almost be perceived as if they were solid, creating an illusion of crowdedness, that the air is filled with 'something'. A conference room full of people, a subway at rush hour or a busy restaurant can feel 'filled up' perhaps even oppressive to someone who can smell but this is something he simply cannot imagine. Smells travel quickly and can hint at what is beyond sight and hearing, at times over great distances. 'Being anosmic I therefore have a more limited horizon of perception. Someone sitting in another room can tell if coffee is being made, if dinner is ready. I don't get any such information from my surroundings.'

Looking back on his life, Lundqvist says that it is his wife who taught him most about smell and tried to make him aware of the world inhabited by those who do have their fifth sense. But this was all trial and error, not the kind of systematic training that occurs naturally as children grow up and learn to take care of their rooms, their living environments, change clothes, negotiate personal hygiene. Sometimes, his wife's remarks can still feel irritating, even unfair, but without them he would never have learned how to behave and shape his decisions to the unwritten rules about smells in human society. 'So I guess I owe it to her that I have been able to act in a socially acceptable way over the years. Looking back, I can't help but wonder how I functioned before meeting her and how we could end up married and having a family!' There are published studies that suggest that anosmics have more problems finding a partner, feel more insecure and have fewer relationships. He tells me, 'Maybe I was just lucky.'

6

Mapping the Nose

Do you like coriander? I love it and will happily use it in cooking, add it to salads or just munch on it fresh. My mother, Mariella, detests it. A wonderful cook (and retired academic with a brain like a planet), she will not countenance its use as an ingredient in any dish let alone consider eating it on its own. Coriander (or cilantro as it is known in the United States) polarises people, so much so that an 'I hate coriander' Facebook page now boasts nearly 300,000 members, has spawned a line of clothing and accessories and haters celebrate their shared loathing each year on 24 February. In 2020, just as the world began to brace for the Covid onslaught, the *Daily Mail* reported Anti-Coriander Day and the article quickly went viral, shared thousands of times and provoking a flood of reader comments from Australia to Zimbabwe. 'I'll celebrate "I hate coriander day" today and every day,' wrote one reader. 'How about founding a new country, coriander-free?' added another.

The earliest scientific study to find out what causes the divisive response sparked by the herb was done with twins in the early 2000s by Charles Wysocki, a behavioural neuroscientist at the Monell Chemical Senses Center in Philadelphia. He found that about 80 per cent of identical twins shared the same preference (or not) for the herb. Fraternal twins who share half their genome, however, agreed only half the time. This suggested strongly that there is a heritable component to whether you are a coriander lover or hater. (If you hold your nose and bite into the leaves, you will barely notice the taste even if it is, for you, the devil's herb.)

In 2012, a California-based consumer genetics firm, 23andMe sent out a survey to 30,000 people asking whether the herb tasted like soap and whether or not they liked it. Researchers then went on to identify two common genetic variants linked to the 'soap' group and follow-up studies confirmed the association. Scientists estimate that up to 14 per cent of people carry this genetic difference, which means that they, like my mother, perceive 'soap' where the great majority savour the tangy, aromatic, slightly peppery 'greenness' of the herb that I adore. The main coriander gene, known as OR6A2, encodes a receptor that is highly sensitive to aldehyde chemicals, the major flavour constituents of the offending herb but which are also often found in soaps and lotions.

Coriander is an intriguing further illustration of the complexity of our sense of smell and the host of factors, including our genes, that govern perception. Equally, what animals and insects perceive and smell is different for each species, much of it shaped by adaptation to the environments in which they live and must try to survive. The detection of food gases by ammonia-seeking soil bacteria or a vulture's ability to detect an animal carcass miles away indicates the vast array of scents registered by different species and how their biosphere has shaped what they are primed to smell, recognise and locate.

Despite these differences, there is also a fundamental same-ness to the way all animals process smells: vertebrates like us absorb the smell first into the nasal mucus, which then takes the odour molecule and attaches it to what is known as an odour-binding protein (OBP), the tiny escort that helps ensure it travels safely through the mucus and onto the receptor. Invertebrates such as insects, spiders and crustaceans behave in a similar way using their antennae, which also contain a viscous fluid, as they absorb the smell and carry it through to their own receptors.

University of Manchester zoologist Professor Matthew Cobb explains that the precise function of these OBPs is still unknown but studies have shown just how important they are in the ecology of some animals. Pandas, for example, have an OBP that works solely with the odours found in bamboo, their sole source of food, while the fly, *Drosophila sechellia*, has an OBP that allows it to seek out the pungent fruit of the Indian mulberry, which has a unique odour and which other competing species are simply unable to recognise. Other OBPs have been found to be respon-sive to humidity or simply to work as chaperones for the odour molecules as they travel towards their receptors.[1]

Anatomists throughout the ages, from Hippocrates in ancient times to the Renaissance and Leonardo da Vinci, attempted to observe, study and document the internal structures of the nose and nasal cavities but it wasn't until the 1820s when the French anatomist and physician Hippolyte Cloquet, elaborating on work done by German colleagues, became the first to identify the vitally important role of the 'escort' mucus in that first instant when we sniff, just prior to recognition of the smell. Cloquet was able to describe the pathway, into the nostrils and back into the spacious cavity where the layer of mucus resides and which he believed acted to slow down the odorant's travel, trapping it and separating it from the air. From there, he suggested it would move upwards to meet with the olfactory nerve and then transmit the message back into the brain.

Physiologists would later embark on various grisly experiments in the 1880s in an effort to try to map this pathway into the brain. One, by the great Viennese scientist Eduard Paulsen, saw him use a human head sawn in half lengthwise, with litmus paper stuck all along the nasal cavities. The head was then put back together and a tube inserted up the nose through which was pumped air sprinkled with ammonia to test for a reaction with the litmus paper. A pig's bladder acting like mock lungs completed the mimicking of the respiration process. Similar experiments with the heads of horses would add knowledge about the passage of odorants towards and into the nasal mucus while the invention and wider use of staining techniques would help identify what we now know to be neural structures. All this slowly added to a more detailed understanding of the olfactory pathway.

The difficulty always lay with odorants' unpredictable nature. Unlike light and sound waves, which are relatively stable stimuli and can be measured and documented, odorants behave very differently depending on how they interact with other smells already in the surrounding air. By the late 1890s, German and American scientists had also embarked on studies to record the myriad responses elicited by the same or similar odorants along with careful observation of the impact and complex interplay between the stimulus itself and how the person perceiving it is feeling at the time.

Eleanor Gamble, an American scientist, was one of the first to work with smell perception in a scientific setting; at the end of the nineteenth century, she observed and reported the effect of fatigue on smell perception and the fact that we filter out some smells while others appear to become less intense when we are exposed to them over a period of time – a phenomenon called habituation. Anyone who wears perfume or aftershave will notice that the scent seems to disappear after a while. Gamble however showed that some odours, such as coumarin and vanilla, have a maximum intensity that simply cannot be made stronger and in fact become unpleasant at higher concentration.[2] Measuring these perceptual changes with any accuracy was difficult and would ultimately lead to the invention of specialist instruments, including the Zwaardemaker olfactometer, a contraption of glass pipes and porous porcelain designed to trap smelly liquids in a bid to measure the intensity of smells and to test responses and their effect more precisely.

*

Theories on olfaction remained as varied as they were unsatisfying. Most between the 1920s and the 1970s suggested some form of vibration of – or between – olfactory cells and the chemical stimulus. Others speculated that it was all about absorption by the mucus membranes followed by an interaction with a chain of enzymes. More disciplines would apply their knowledge to try to unravel the question and chemists joined physicists who joined physiologists and clinicians in the race to find rules that might explain odorants' behaviour through their structures (studies that became known as SORs or Structure-Odour-Rules). Ultimately,

the sheer multiplicity of alternatives that make up single odorants frustrated attempts to build hard-and-fast rules for smell and
failed to unlock the magic code for how the nose smells particular
molecules. Lock-and-key models also proved to be inadequate
while the idea that the olfactory epithelium might contain specific
areas allowing it to be mapped for odours was explored right into
the 1970s.

Ideas and hypotheses abounded but unlike vision, which was
already a booming field of neuroscience, both well funded and
well supported, olfaction remained the poor cousin, despite the
fact that nobody could say much beyond the fact that smells
were brought by individual molecules, which carried their own,
specific scent.

By the end of the 1970s, stung by the lack of funding for
olfactory studies, a small group of American researchers and
a handful of their European counterparts decided it was time
to join forces and advocate for funding as a united group. They
established an international group, known as the Association for
Chemoreception Sciences (AChemS) and launched a concerted,
systematic campaign to unravel the molecular secrets of the fifth
sense in the mid 1980s. Ann-Sophie Barwich describes the subsequent launch of the first 'hardcore' cellular and molecular biology
research in several laboratories around the world, from Germany
and Israel to the United States:

> With growing insight into a common mechanism of molec-
> ular communication, it stood to reason that smell could be
> subject to the same general principles governing the other
> processes . . . a key but missing piece of the puzzle involved

the membrane receptors that started this whole molecular gateway.

＊

Linda Buck is the pioneering scientist who in 1991, together with Richard Axel at Columbia University in New York, worked to identify the family of genes that allows us humans to detect and distinguish smells. Their work eventually earned them a Nobel Prize in 2004. Today, chemosensory and cognitive scientists often talk about the history of olfactory research as if there were two eras, 'before and after Buck', so enormous was the find and so significant its impact.

As a post-doctoral student working in Axel's Howard Hughes Medical Institute, Buck had become obsessed with the mysterious and elusive olfactory receptors. Fellow neuroscientists had spent decades trying to unravel the visual system and were well on the way to cracking its codes. By 1986, the three main colour receptors, for blue, green and red light, had been discovered, while the combination code that lets us perceive the different wavelengths that make up light and identify the colours of the rainbow was also understood. Yet, at this time, the small group of scientists who were researching the Cinderella sense knew only that odour molecules bind to nasal cells before sending signals to the olfactory bulb and the brain. Exactly what receptors did they bind with? At that point, they had no real idea. There appeared to be a baffling variety and number of recognisable smells and it was envisaged that perhaps it worked like our visual system, and a handful of main receptors worked together with shared or overlapping sensitivities to account for the myriad sensibilities.

Buck was working on the nervous system of a sea slug when in 1985 a paper on the olfactory system grabbed her imagination and changed her life: 'It was a publication . . . that discussed potential mechanisms underlying odour detection. This was the first time I had ever thought about olfaction and I was fascinated. How could humans and other mammals detect 10,000 or more odorous chemicals, and how could nearly identical chemicals generate different odour perceptions?'

In Buck's mind, this was the monumental puzzle she had been looking for as it offered an unparalleled diversity problem. The first step to solving the conundrum, she decided, was to work out how odorants are initially detected in the nose and this would require finding odorant receptors, a class of molecules that scientists had proposed might exist but which had yet to be found.

As everyone else who had gone looking for the receptors had failed miserably, Buck suggested that she would search instead for the gene that encodes them. She also said she would limit her hunt by working the research process around three assumptions. First, she expected that this would be a multi-gene family; second, that they'd be expressed only in the olfactory epithelium, and third, that the proteins that they encode might well be similar to the receptor proteins we have in our eyes. Using all three of these basic suppositions meant that the size of the search was greatly reduced. Richard Axel would later tell reporters that Buck's brave assumptions saved them 'years of drudgery'.

Buck recalled that she worked on the genome of rats for two and a half years, working fifteen-hour days before she had the breakthrough that would so dramatically jolt the world of sensory physiology.

The Nobel Prize would recognise Buck not just for identifying the existence of receptor genes in rats – detailed in the landmark paper the duo published in 1991[3] – but for the huge body of work she produced in the decade that followed. This included the discovery of about a thousand different olfactory genes in rats – way more than she or anyone had expected – and similar families of odorant receptors in many other vertebrate species, ranging from fish to humans. To provide some perspective, the mammalian genome contains somewhere around 20,000 genes with a pretty significant percentage of them devoted exclusively to being able to smell.

Buck and her team found that each olfactory receptor cell possesses just one type of odorant receptor although each receptor can detect a limited number of odorant substances. This means our olfactory receptor cells are highly specialised for a few odours. However it is when these cells send signals to distinct tiny areas of the olfactory bulb, known as glomeruli, that the magic happens because when information from several olfactory cells is combined, it forms a pattern. Our perception of a smell, its identification and later recall or memory, is derived from these patterns of olfactory receptor recognition – all of it processed by our brains. Therefore, it isn't a case of one key for one lock (one odorant per receptor) but rather, that different smell molecules activate different combinations of olfactory receptors, thereby sending different signals to the brain. The unprecedented size and diversity of the family of genes at last went some way to explaining mammals' ability to detect such a vast array of diverse smells as well as identify that very similar chemicals can also have distinct odours.

Our olfactory receptors were later found to form part of an even bigger family of proteins known as G-protein-coupled receptors (GCPRs), which are inherent to an array of functions in our bodies, from immune response right through to vision. They help us by behaving a little as though they are taking part in a relay race, creating a chemical response within each cell, which then sparks an electrical charge if enough receptors have been turned on along the way.

Writing not long after the award, Buck's friend and fellow neuroscientist, Stuart Firestein, observed that her findings immediately opened an endless, new array of research possibilities to their olfactory colleagues. Ideas about different types of coding mechanisms that had been bandied about for decades could now either be dismissed very quickly or re-embraced for further research. For example, the possibility that colour vision might be analogous to smell and that there might be only a handful of 'primary' receptors tuned to so-called 'primary' odorants in the way colour works could now be jettisoned thanks to Buck and Axel unmasking hundreds of odorant receptors when it was known that there are only three colour receptors.

As I became familiar with Buck's remarkable finds, I was struck by her need – even after winning the Nobel Prize – to defend her choice of the olfactory system for her research work:

> Even some science journalists have asked me what diseases this olfaction research might cure. I think a lot of people don't realise that basic science generates the sort of fundamental information that's required to understand things like disease processes and disease prevention. There's also

a lot of cross-talk between fields, where research into the sense of taste might for some unexpected reason prove to be crucial to understanding, say, cancer.

Three decades later, her doubts seemed even more poignant because the race to explain the global olfactory devastation and epidemic of smell loss caused by the Covid virus would simply have been impossible without her game-changing findings. (And the world's coriander haters wouldn't have a scientific excuse to demand that the devil's herb be kept off their dinner plates.)

7

The Taste of Rotting Water

I'm waking and I'm trying to wash the sewage out
of my mouth. It isn't easy to do . . .[1]

About ten days before the UK was put into Covid lock-down, British playwright Sir David Hare was holed up in an airless cutting room in London's West End. He'd received a call asking him to come in to help with Episode Two of *Roadkill,* his BBC thriller about a politician haunted by skeletons in the closet. 'It's about a Conservative politician who is forward-looking, intelligent, charismatic and popular. It's not based on anyone in real life,' he quipped.

TV scriptwriters, it seems, are convinced that when it comes to four-part series, the second episode is always the most difficult and this one, observed Hare, had 'severe bruising from a producer's pile on . . . a bugger's muddle'. Convinced the script would benefit from his steadying, mature hand, Hare joined the director, Michael Keillor, and an editor to work on fresh cuts. Over several hours, as complex machinery hummed and whirred in the windowless warmth, the trio sweated over the script, sharing tea, biscuits – and fetid air. The following day, Keillor rang Hare not to tell him that the edits had gone well but that on returning home that night he'd collapsed and the next morning he could neither move nor breathe. He had contracted Covid and Hare would shortly follow suit.

What unfolded over the following fifteen days is recounted by Hare in a riveting monologue he would title *Beat the Devil* and which would be performed at London's Bridge Theatre during the brief summer respite before the onset of the second wave. The play was critically acclaimed, as was Ralph Fiennes' performance delivering Hare's 'raw, acid, furious' rant from his sickbed. The terror of contracting Covid in the earliest days of the pandemic and his white-hot rage at the Tory government's dithering before ordering the first lockdown put paid to any fears that audiences might avoid the show due to Covid fatigue. Instead, it became emblematic of the return of live theatre to the capital.

I bought the script, eager to read any shared experiences and was immediately struck by the monologue's wry gallows humour. There is a very funny moment when he describes his wife, Nicole, climbing on top of him to keep him warm as he shivered through the fevers: 'My wife doesn't seem to have grasped the notion of social distancing.' However, what stopped me in my tracks was his arresting opening lines, which described waking up one morning to the inescapable taste of sewage in his mouth: 'Everything tastes of sewage. When I go to the tap at five in the morning and drink fresh water, all I can taste is sewage.'

What is extraordinary, in retrospect, is that while the critics all referred to Hare's vivid depiction of fatigue, aches, teeth-rattling chills, temperatures and drenching sweats, none mentioned what was clearly an experience of the smell distortions that can accompany olfactory damage and that we would soon learn would become a hallmark of Covid.

Intrigued by his experience, I contacted Sir David to ask if he could try to reconstruct what he could recall of the week preceding the onset of his smell and taste distortions and if he had had any inkling that he might have become anosmic and lost his sense of smell first. 'Is the word for what I had anosmia?' he replied.

> I don't know. I never lost my sense of taste or smell. The problem was that my mouth tasted – to use the correct word – of shit, and everything I ate tasted of shit too. I could not get rid of the taste.
>
> I went to bed on March 21, but things only got bad on Friday 27 when I thought I felt better, so I made chicken with bean sprouts. It tasted vile. That night I began vomiting and having diarrhoea, and the real nightmare began – wild fevers, hot and cold. What was most alarming was that when I went to the tap for water to clean out my mouth, it tasted of sewage. It did nothing to clean my mouth – nor did toothpaste, nor Listerine.

Unable to stomach the nightmare taste, he stopped eating altogether and dropped seven or eight kilos in a week because nothing would stay down.

> My wife would give me clear soups, but I would vomit them an hour later. I assumed the bad taste came from

dehydration, so I drank as much water as I could, but it still tasted bad. I was too tired to eat and revolted at the thought of food.

The only thing I could keep down was hot water with honey and ginger. It did taste good – and to this day the memory of it is very sweet and cheering to me.

Then, on the sixteenth day of his illness, just as suddenly as it had appeared, the ugly sewage taste disappeared. He remembers waking up to a ravenous hunger – and to his wife's utter surprise.

My wife refused to believe it and thought I would just vomit again. But I didn't. I smelt the air that morning and it no longer smelt of sewage. I have no idea why.

Sir David would turn out to be one of the lucky ones, his experience of parosmia, while violent in combination with the virus, was short and sharp. As every nation ravaged by Covid would soon learn, the most common trajectory for those struck with a relatively mild dose of the virus is smell loss, followed several weeks later by the distortions. But at that early point in the pandemic, when anosmia, let alone such strange olfactory disruptions, was yet to be recognised as a symptom, physicians told me that it is likely that the British playwright was one of the very first known cases of the epidemic of smell distortions that would afflict hundreds of thousands of people just two months later.

I remember that by early summer I had begun to perceive inklings of smells, so faint they made me think of ghost fragrances:

the memory of freshly picked rosemary when I crushed it between my fingernails, a waft of jasmine in a neighbour's garden and one day, my favourite perfume, Le Labo's Santal 33 (leathery, tobacco-y, musky) yielded a whisper of itself. My diary shows that in the following days I fried onions and lashings of garlic and cumin together and nearly cried because my nose was oblivious to what my brain knew to be the most intoxicating and appetising of cooking aromas. At that point I couldn't smell coffee as coffee at all but one evening I forgot that anosmia had ruined the experience of eating chocolate and bit into what I now assume must have been a soft-centre filled with artificial coffee essence. That, strangely, was perceptible in the way I remembered coffee to be.

Then, just as my personal olfactory desert seemed to be yielding the occasional fruit – and psychological encouragement – my sensory world tilted and seemed to become infused with charcoal. The smell of burning appeared the day after we'd spent a socially distanced evening with friends, hunched around a fire pit for warmth. The all-pervasive smell of campfire smoke that has to be washed out of your hair, clothes and skin fixed resolutely into my nose and brain, inescapable, oppressive and, at times, terrifying. I began to pester my husband and daughter, asking several times a day if they could smell burning and it took some time for my instincts to accept that we were not in imminent danger. It was a period of being on hyper-alert and yet once, when I did leave a tea towel too close to the stove, singeing it to a black crust, I failed to register that as real. I was experiencing what would later be described by some researchers as a 'smell lock' and in some ways I felt fortunate because what others were going through in ever-increasing numbers seemed far, far worse.

The most common descriptors, like Sir David Hare's, referred to sewage, rotting fruit or the stench of garbage bags left in the sun but many others recounted the most unexpected perceptions – of stale vanilla stench, of mouths ravaged by the taste of licking metal or inhaling nail polish remover, of burnt chemicals, swallowed pool water, snorting mouldy garlic or even onions blended in with milk. Some people thought it was their toothbrush and changed it for a new one as they scrubbed away at the taste and smell. Others, like my friend, became convinced one of their children had urinated in the house.

When one woman in America posted the question: How would you describe Covid taste/smell?, within hours it elicited nearly 400 answers including my personal favourite, described vividly by Gina M, a woman in Manchester who wrote that hers was like 'mouldy, peppery cloth'. Karina C reported that during her anosmia phase everything smelled or tasted like day-old tap water, but with parosmia, 'It felt like someone grabbed a handful of garden weeds and brushed my teeth with it, shoved it up my nose, pushed back into my throat and then left it there.' 'It smells like Covid,' observed Amanda Finch in Lancashire to a resounding chorus of approval. 'It has its own awful smell, unique to everyone. Something that I recognise and can't place at the same time. It's bloody awful and annoying!'[2] When I fell on a post from a nurse in California who was haunted by the smell of campfire smoke, I was taken aback by my own sense of relief at not being alone and understood just how important it can be to share experiences, to test your own reality with others but particularly so when medicine had yet to catch up and provide answers.

Dr Duika Burges Watson, a British-Australian social scientist with the Population Health Sciences Institute at the University of Newcastle in the UK, is probably one of only a handful of specialists around the world who would immediately have recognised David Hare's early, bewildering experience with parosmia. Her work explores the complex relationship between food and well-being. In 2014, she had launched the first major, long-term investigation of the eating difficulties experienced by survivors of head and neck cancers. As compassionate as she is dynamic and driven, Burges Watson recalls that one of her earliest meetings during what would become a six-year study was with a woman who had suffered terrible smell distortions in the wake of her chemotherapy. 'She had literally divided her house in half, physically, because she couldn't stand the smell of her partner's cooking,' she told me. 'At that point in time, in the field I was working in, nobody knew the term parosmia, nobody was familiar with it, we certainly didn't know how to help her.'

By the time Covid-induced anosmia sufferers began to report parosmia in numbers, Burges Watson had already been working closely as an adviser with UK charity AbScent and its founder Chrissi Kelly, helping people affected by olfactory disorders explore and find new ways to enjoy eating. 'When we started seeing the Facebook posts about the smell of poo, sewage, the horror about coffee, which seems to be a universal one, we knew straight away that something was going on. We were suddenly faced with this huge population with parosmia and decided it was important to document it. This was such a unique moment for us to bring this little-known condition to light.'[3]

Strange as it may seem, Burges Watson told me that it is not uncommon for water – which people usually describe as having no taste – to be a trigger for parosmia. Two years before the global outbreak of smell distortions, she had been asked to work on a panel for Northumbria Water, which, paradoxically, while managing the least-treated natural water supply in the UK, receives more consumer complaints about its taste than any other authority. 'Bizarrely, they get their water from four different sources and, depending on the season, it might come from different reservoirs or the Derwent river but every time the sources change and reach people's taps they get complaints. They wanted to work out strategies to manage this.'

Water does in fact have a taste, usually flavoured by the environment that surrounds it, and it is treated only when it requires purification. In most cases, natural occurrences such as benign algae growth don't warrant the addition of chemicals. 'Further south in the UK, for example, water is chlorinated because it is so heavily treated and yet people don't complain because they're used to it. I realised that what was happening in Northumbria says a lot about habituation: we get used to smells or flavours and feel something isn't right and complain when these change.'

As Kelly and Burges Watson encountered more and more Covid-induced parosmia sufferers, it became clear that not all of them found water disgusting in the way Sir David Hare and many others did.[4] People often described the 'smell' of water as chemical – like chlorine or pool water – or sweet and sickly – like a dirty dishrag or even like the seaside. Instead, they appeared to have suddenly become ultra-sensitive or intolerant of particular hints or 'notes' perceived immediately as they filled a glass with water. 'For a lot of people, that hyper-sensitivity can be over-whelming even when they're doing other things such as washing their hands or even taking a shower,' Burges Watson recalled. 'This is because when water is heated, volatile odours in the water are released into the air and the smell they perceive reaches them much more easily.'

In Florida, seventeen-year-old Evelyn T described her paros-mia and distress with extraordinary clarity for her age in a note published by the BBC: 'It's as though an invisible hand came out of nowhere, distorting my nose and tongue. The most unbearable is tap water. Showering, rinsing dishes, brushing my teeth, washing my face and many more daily encounters are now repulsive and unbearable. Living in a world where tap water smells putrid has been one of the hardest things I've ever gone through,' she wrote.

By late summer, Burges Watson became so puzzled by the growing numbers of people unable to stomach tap water that she decided to dig around and find out if anyone had been working on or researching the taste and flavour of good ol' acqua pura in more normal times. Her research, she told me, led her to 'the amazing Gary Burlingame', an American environmental scientist who had done some really interesting work on how to 'name' the odours in water. He had also written a detective-style memoir about his journey through the sensory world of water entitled *Earthy, with a Hint of Cucumber*. Burlingame is also Director of Philadelphia Water's Bureau of Laboratory Services and Burges Watson decided to approach him to ask if he would help put together a survey of water companies in the US, Canada and UK: 'We wanted to see if they've had unusual patterns of com-plaints about parosmia and water. Researchers will also work with the University of Reading's Dr Jane Parker to see if there are more complaints about particular water sources and, if so, that might help them identify the molecular triggers for the parosmia response to water.'

*

Burges Watson's agile response to exploring new smell and taste problems was born of a fateful moment in the United States several years earlier when she and an oncologist colleague had been paddling a canoe during a river trip hosted by a medical conference. As they paddled and chatted, she'd told him about her PhD and research interests in carrageenan, a red, edible seaweed farmed for its thickening and stabilising properties, while he'd confided that he feared his work curing head and neck cancers only led to making patients' lives intolerable.

The conversation about cancer patients' struggles with food and altered eating had a cathartic effect on Burges Watson. She scoured the medical literature only to find that while most cancer patients battled ongoing weight and appetite loss, there was no consistent methodology to help address their quality of life, let alone understand what scientists call 'food hedonics' and exactly what it is that makes food enjoyable to eat. Determined to address the gap in research, Burges Watson pulled together a team of seven colleagues, including one who was both a cancer survivor and researcher, and began to follow twenty-five patients and their partners in a bid to understand the physical and emotional impact of losing the ability to eat well.[5]

The paper was peer-reviewed and published in 2018 and, as an anosmic, I found reading it moving in a way I had not expected. Here were subjects cleared of their cancer but terrified of choking and subsequently too frightened to eat; participants plagued by the lack of saliva, which turned many much-loved dishes and drinks into painful, gritty, burning experiences; hopeful subjects walking into restaurants visualising their favourite curry only to describe the heart-sinking disappointment of smelling and tasting absolutely nothing. One reported that even the need to eat slowly and carefully due to throat damage meant it had become impossible to eat socially any more: '[It's] a big thing and all because once your food starts to go cold, it's even harder to get it down. I'm going to have to tube feed, yeah, I'm just getting fed up trying to eat, it takes so long, it's just a chore.' As with parosmics, food had effectively morphed from a pleasure, shared with others, to a tiring necessity devoid of any sensory joy.

The cumulative effect of this tiring and labour-intensive relationship with food dramatically changed both their social life and sense of identity because as much as they mourned the loss of taste and flavour, they also mourned the inclusion and feeling of belonging that food offers most of us, even if we don't think much about it. Burges Watson's work paved the way for the launch of the Altered Eating Research Network, which continues to study and develop strategies for people who struggle to feed themselves in the wake of diseases including cancer, Sjögren's syndrome (an immune disease that results in dry eyes and an impossibly dry mouth) and brain injuries.

Indeed, as the parosmia epidemic created by Covid swept the world, Burges Watson found herself in the very special position of being able to offer some solace – and practical survival strategies – to those unable to stomach food or water. Chief among them is to focus on the other senses, add texture to your food, make it look, feel and sound good for you. Bland and bold foods have been shown to work best for those with parosmia: mushroom and tofu for example are often more palatable than cooked meats. Cold foods are easier to manage than hot ones, as lower temperatures reduce the evaporation of aroma compounds. Burges Watson warns that there is no magic formula because everyone's experience of parosmia is different. Talking to others about what worked for them and pushing yourself to become your own detective for the foods you can stomach is important.

'I've thought a lot about that first woman we spoke to all those years ago who couldn't even stand the scent of her partner's skin let alone cooking smells: we had no idea how much she was really struggling then. If I knew then what we know now I'd have been able to help more.'

8

Wake up and Smell the Coffee

Increasingly intrigued by the vagaries of smell distortions, I decided it was time to explore the laboratory of Jane Parker, Associate Professor of Flavour Chemistry at the University of Reading and founder of the world-renowned Flavour Centre. She has made it her life's business to study the compounds that are responsible for what our noses and tongues perceive when they work together. Chatting over Zoom one morning in the middle of the second lockdown, I asked Dr Parker to explain a little about her work with flavour, which is ultimately what we actually experience when our olfactory system and tongue interact.

Taste, in Europe at least, was always thought to be about what the tongue alone perceives: sweet, sour, salt and bitter until the Japanese 'umami' – or savoury taste – was added to the list. This was the work of Kikunae Ikeda, a Professor at Tokyo Imperial University who discovered in 1908 that glutamate was responsible for making kombu seaweed palatable, indeed delicious. He noticed that *kombu dashi* (broth) was quite different from the other tastes and named it umami. (Many researchers since have argued that there are other possibilities related to pungent spices but let's stick with the five main ones for now.)

Dr Parker explained:

In comparison with the five tastes, there are at least 10,000 different compounds with distinct aromas. Each of these is likely to have a distinct set of aroma receptors in our noses so that each of us perceives or experiences smells differently. Furthermore, our sensitivity to some of these compounds is extreme: dilute a swimming pool full of water with one drop of a sulphur compound for example and it can still produce a distinct meaty smell.

The main instrument used in Dr Parker's laboratory is the Gas Chromatography-Olfactometer (GC-O), which uses inert gases and 30 metres of a fine-as-hair fused silica capillary to help researchers separate aroma compounds into their molecular components:

We take an extract of the aroma, which is the smell you get when you put your nose in, let's say, a cup of coffee. This is what we call the headspace. Coffee has thousands of compounds in it but just 20 or 30 are very important. We tease them apart, look at what they are and what they smell like individually.

Our biological noses, says Dr Parker, can beat the very best laboratory instruments, even when it comes to detecting the tiniest amounts of these substances. Occasionally her work has become even trickier when the amounts fall below the levels detectable by the instruments or when odours are masked by other more abundant, if perhaps less powerful, compounds.

While much of the centre's research is for the food industry, working to tease out optimum flavours in manufacturing, in mid 2019 Dr Parker embarked on an entirely different path of olfactory study, thanks to a chance meeting with Chrissi Kelly. The AbScent founder had been invited to speak at a conference in Amsterdam by Dr Craig Duckham, a leading British flavour scientist who had become intrigued by her experience of anosmia and smell distortions during a Twitter exchange. Kelly agreed and delivered a lively talk to explain the strange olfactory disturbance that can suddenly turn an array of normally pleasant food odours into unbearable, indescribable stenches. Kelly had lost her sense of smell in 2012 after a sinus infection and a year into her recovery suffered terrible parosmia. It had turned the pleasure of eating and drinking into a nightmare for months on end and while it had passed for her, she became adamant that olfactory dysfunctions, largely unrecognised or underestimated by doctors for too long, should be brought into the public spotlight and was hell-bent on finding evidence-based ways to explain and alleviate her fellow parosmics' suffering.

Over the years, she had gathered detailed information from fellow sufferers and had put together and even painted a watercolour 'periodic table-style' graphic to illustrate the groups of foods that patients reported were often triggers for the syndrome.

> After I spoke, Jane came up to me and said, 'You know what? I think I know what the problem is.' I had ended

my talk and PowerPoint presentation with a drawing of Sherlock Holmes' Dr Watson, saying, 'I say Holmes, why are these foods such a dashed nuisance to people with parosmia?' Holmes replied, 'The answer, Watson, lies with the food scientists.'

Kelly laughed, recalling the exchange. Dr Parker continued the story:

Chrissi had gathered some very interesting information from the social media group she'd set up for people with parosmia. Coffee, chocolate, meat were repeat offenders, others mentioned onion, garlic, eggs. As a flavour chemist, I recognised immediately that the most troublesome foods they reported all share a small group of aroma chemicals that are fairly similar.

What was particularly interesting is that I knew these foods to contain aroma molecules with some of the lowest odour-thresholds known . . . I felt it was quite possible that it may well be these that were triggering the distortions.

Parosmia patients often find it almost impossible to find the words to describe what it is like to live with a syndrome that turns much-loved foods into reeking hunks of rotting meat or worse. Some sufferers lose vast amounts of weight, incapable of conquering the smell-induced nausea, while others find themselves gravitating to the foods that fail to trigger distortion such as salty, crunchy crisps but which ultimately limit dietary choice and lead to eating just to feel full, with subsequent weight gain.

Immediately enthused by their potential new line of inquiry, the challenge for Kelly was to try to find enough parosmia sufferers willing to volunteer their noses to Dr Parker's GC-O. By October that year, Parker had signed on an associate researcher in Kelly and she had managed to deliver fifteen volunteers, most of whom had become parosmic after viral illness or brain injury but all of whom were happy to be put through their paces in the Flavour Centre laboratory. Dr Parker found 'normosmic' fellow researchers and students to enrol as the control group.

The first round of research in the last months of 2019 – just months before Covid would envelop the world – was groundbreaking: the GC-O was used to break down the aroma of coffee into its myriad components to determine which of the molecules present triggered the immediate recoil and sense of disgust. Dr Parker settled on coffee because it contains a thousand or so volatile molecules, among them sulphur compounds, for example, which are responsible for the stench of rotten eggs. The combination of all these different chemicals, dancing together in particular proportions and patterns, is what produces the overall delightful 'aroma profile' of freshly brewed coffee or an espresso bubbling on the stove.

It's a morning ritual shared by many cultures to shake off the torpor of the night and even those who don't like drinking the stuff will often say they enjoy its smell: nutty, toasty, perhaps a little smoky. I've sometimes wondered if the bitter taste of coffee is slightly disappointing after the expectation elicited by the joy of its aroma. And yet, many parosmia sufferers say coffee is the first culprit they notice, producing an unrecognisable stench, different from anything they have ever experienced before. During that first round of experiments, the distorted smell turned out to be so alien that Parker and her researchers were forced to use the simple label 'new coffee' as a descriptor for the olfactory experience her subjects were reporting.

I asked Dr Parker, if coffee aroma comprises so many volatile molecules, including some sulphurs that produce bad smells, why don't we respond to them all? 'We think that it is to do with the dose . . . at low levels it might be perceived as pleasant but as concentration increases that is when it can get revolting,' she told me.

In normal noses, the neurones fire when the receptors detect their own particular chemicals are present, sending information to the brain via the olfactory bulb. It is this pattern – that lovely dance of neurones firing – that allows our brain to identify the entire aroma picture. Dr Parker and her olfactory clinician colleagues suspected that in parosmia, this ability to interpret patterns is disrupted: 'If you knock out enough receptors and have only a few working, as we think might be happening with parosmia, then it just gives you an incomplete signal to the brain.'

Another possible cause might be the loss of a group of very specific receptors that accompany specific molecules, perhaps tricking the brain into perceiving some compounds (such as the stinky sulphur ones) alone. Mixed in together, some smelly substances temper or add to a fragrance, a little bit of alchemy that perfumers have known about for a long time. For example, two of the more common compounds used in perfumery, indole and skatole, smell faecal in high concentration but at low doses with selected others they're rounded and pleasant odours.

Another hypothesis was that the distortion was occurring at an even more complex level, the result of an interaction with receptors that are excited by some molecules but shut down by others. If that perfect balance is lost, perhaps so is coffee's harmonious aroma profile. The picture was further complicated by the observation that while some hideous odours are perfectly preserved by the nose of a parosmia sufferer, many reported that what they knew normally as horrible smells were no longer recognisable nor, at times, quite as disgusting.

Dr Parker and Chrissi Kelly's earliest, first attempts to explore parosmia in the laboratory unfolded with just a handful of enthusiastic and dedicated volunteers. Would they be enough?

And then along came Covid.

PART 2

9

Puppysnot and Froonkle

The day dawned chilly and clear in Umbria, the hilly, forested region of Italy often referred to as the country's green heart. On 12 March 2020, inside the Gubbio-Gualdo Tadino hospital, about 50 kilometres north of Perugia, ENT physician Dr Puya Dehgani-Mobaraki was already at work preparing for a busy morning's surgery ahead. In Italy, it is national custom to grab a quick breakfast 'cornetto' and coffee at a cafe before work, and the hospital canteen observed this ritual, fragrant with freshly baked pastries. The noise of the espresso machine was dulled only by the chatter of colleagues standing at the bar waiting to throw back the shiny black contents of the tiny cup like a shot of vodka.

When a colleague mentioned the smell of a croissant burning in the cafe toaster, Dr Dehgani-Mobaraki was surprised that he had not noticed, but dismissed it as he headed off downstairs to prepare for patients. It was only then that he realised he could not smell the alcohol-based disinfectants or the powerful bleach in the ammonia-based detergents used in operating theatres: 'I put my nose right into the ammonia but there was nothing. Nothing,' he recalled.

The first case in Italy of Covid-19 had been confirmed in Rome on 31 January, traced to two Chinese tourists who had tested positive soon after arriving from Beijing. The first confirmed death, a seventy-eight-year-old man in the Veneto region, occurred three weeks later, on 22 February. As Dr Dehgani-Mobaraki finished with his last patient that March afternoon, the Italian prime minister, Giuseppe Conte, announced the extension of quarantine from Lombardy in the north to cover the entire nation, placing more than 60 million people into a state of emergency and total lockdown.

The following day, perplexed by the sudden onset of smell loss, Dr Dehgani-Mobaraki decided that because it had occurred in the midst of a new respiratory virus pandemic, it might be wise to email ENT friends and colleagues around the world to alert them to what he was experiencing.

At 2.35 p.m. on Saturday 14 March he sent a group email to his network of rhinology physicians around the world, including to Professor Claire Hopkins, President of the British Rhinological Society. It read, in part: 'Two days ago I suddenly lost my sense of smell and 90 per cent of taste . . . starting to worry . . . I would ask you to ask this question to all patients, as this at least in Italy is not a parameter.'

'We were all doing endoscopies, tracheotomies in difficult cases . . . I really wanted to tell people to be careful,' he told me. 'Two days later, I heard that one of my endoscopy patients had been hospitalised with Covid and died just twenty-four hours later. I am sure I got it from him.'

Dr Dehgani-Mobaraki would spend more than a week fearing he had Covid but he was unable to convince the hospital authorities that he should be isolating, based on his loss of smell alone. 'Thankfully no one was infected,' he recalled, clearly still uncomfortable at the memory. 'As ENT physicians we know that this can happen with some viral illnesses but I felt this was different. I had been wearing masks nine hours a day and I was also starting to worry because my colleagues scattered all around Italy confirmed that many of them were in the same condition and that many patients were presenting with the same symptoms.'

Scientists and physicians are understandably sceptical of anecdotal reports untested by rigorous methodology. However, the young ENT doctor's experience, lived first hand, had added a new gravitas to flurrying rumours that something strange was unfolding in the noses of Covid patients. Young, bright and an energetic advocate for his medical specialty, Dr Dehgani-Mobaraki had also founded Naso Sano ('healthy nose' in Italian), a non-profit research and educational organisation in Italy. His was the first informal medical alert warning about anosmia as a potential signpost of Covid infection and it sent a powerful ripple of concern around the international network of physicians in his field.

'If someone is trusted then his colleagues will say, "Okay, it might be a reality,"' he recalled from his office as we chatted on Zoom one late afternoon. 'I can tell you that if it wasn't for the internet we would have been maybe fifteen days later and, in a pandemic, fifteen days can mean a lot.'

●

'Puppysnot' is the Reddit username of a thirty-something female lawyer from London. Her feisty profile reads 'Fighting for her clients. Wearing sexy mini-skirts & being self-reliant.' But late on the night of 21 March 2020, a week after Dr Mobaraki's email and just two days before the UK entered its first lockdown, the normally autonomous lawyer needed help – or at the very least some answers. Just after 11.30 p.m. she sent out the following post:

> Recovered from Covid-19 and now have no sense of taste or smell – does anyone know when (if) it will come back? . . . I can only taste hot, cold or extremely salty flavours. I can't smell anything. I'm trying to eat to stay healthy but everything tastes like nothing.

It took just eight minutes for someone to answer. 'Froonkle' had endured a particularly bad case of the flu, or so they thought, in the week before Christmas:

> Worst I've ever felt in my life, all the symptoms were very similar to Covid-19. I lost my sense of smell and taste and for some reason the smell of vinegar made me gag.

Puppysnot was still awake, saw the reply and went to her kitchen to retrieve a bottle of vinegar and test Froonkle's experience: 'I just tried smelling vinegar and I can't smell anything sadly,' she reported back just on midnight.

Despite the late hour, other comments followed quickly. 'Davotoula' had experienced mild symptoms and lost his sense of smell on day three: 'Still not back on day six,' he wrote. So too 'Prophetess', who had no symptoms but was on day eleven of having no sense of smell or taste: 'Has anyone else recovered? I'm starting to worry.' Not all were convinced. 'Borisbemyguide' said a loss of smell was common after the flu while 'Mambafan4life' was sceptical, insisting it was probably sinusitis: 'I had this once . . . call your health service. Not every symptom is necessarily coronavirus.' But the response was overwhelmingly from those who had suddenly lost their sense of smell and were bewildered they could perceive absolutely nothing. Significantly, nobody reported nasal congestion.

Later that day Puppysnot's thread was being read across the Atlantic. 'Hey, I'm from NYC and tested positive,' wrote 'wdrub' before detailing his experience as a healthcare worker. His smell had returned but 'very oddly there's like a chemical taste to some foods. If I hold it to my face I can absolutely smell what it really is. Shrimp, garlic, lime and lemon. But it's very strange to have this chemical smell masking the genuine scent.' 'Timmah612' chimed in from Florida: 'I used to love cooking but I can't even smell what I'm doing any more, much less taste for proper flavour. My one true passion is suddenly gone.'

Puppysnot had gone to bed in London by the time 'duck_duck_goose' posted from China. An expatriate English-language teacher working in Hubei province, the heart of the pandemic, she had gone down with Covid much earlier, on 25 January, two days after swathes of the country were locked down. Although her symptoms were minor, she and her husband had also both suddenly lost their sense of smell. The doctors they had consulted locally insisted anosmia was not a symptom and, in desperation, she too posted a similar question online, only to have it removed by unseen moderators. Was there any news she could access, she asked?

No one had an answer.

✦

As Britain settled into its own first, anxiety-ridden weeks of a national lockdown, the internet was rife with worry about smell loss. Conversations about 'nose blindness' dominated discussion groups and consternation was growing about GPs' dismissal of the symptom and health authorities' refusal to take anosmia seriously. There were moments of levity – 'my poop smells like pineapple' – but, in the main, a flurry of fear, confusion and anxiety about the loss of a sense added to the terror of Covid.

As the number of anosmics grew, the realities of its impact on day-to-day life became clearer. Parents couldn't smell their babies' dirty nappies and worried about unwittingly leaving them unchanged; men feared not being able to detect their own body odour and the impact on their partners, and many lamented the loss of taste and joy in food that only added to the isolation of being trapped at home. One woman revealed she had detected a gas leak that her partner simply couldn't smell. Another man reported taste-testing the contents of his girlfriend's kitchen spice rack, including a spoonful of cinnamon that tasted of nothing: 'I still recognise salty, sweet and spicy food so I've just been dumping salt on my meals or a bucket-load of chillies.'

'DrDan' had lost his sense of smell as a child: 'You get used to it,' he offered, in a well-meaning attempt to reassure. 'Don't think I will,' retorted 'GJAllrelius' angrily, who said she relied on meditation and Chinese green tea to help her cope: 'My passion is the Gongfu tea preparation. It's a skill of intensively focused ability and discernment of tasting. I would rather lose both my legs than my ability to taste/smell.'

'Is the anosmia permanent?' asked 'vegan-zombie', prompting a Los Angeles ear, nose and throat specialist, Dr Rami Abdou, to enter the conversation. He and another ENT colleague, Dr Geoffrey Trenkle, posted tips to help Covid sufferers make sense of symptoms that health services were yet to recognise.

'Since we are so early in the coronavirus pandemic, we don't have the data yet to know how long anosmia will last or whether it could possibly be permanent,' he wrote, adding that some patients who had become anosmic through viral illness had taken up to two years to recover fully.

This prognosis did little to calm growing anxiety in cyberspace.

❀

On 31 March, Dr Hendrik Streeck, head virologist at the University of Bonn in Germany announced the results of a first community-based study of the coronavirus. Weeks before, Streeck and his research team had begun to monitor 1,000 residents of the city's Heinsberg district, dubbed Germany's Wuhan by the media as it was the country's worst-hit area. Their aim was to try to understand and map how the Covid virus spreads and create a blueprint for its containment. In fact, Streeck had started by using forty doctoral students to conduct house-to-house interviews with 100 infected residents, taking swabs from door handles, mobile phones, television remote controls and even samples of toilet water. On 16 March, asked by a *Frankfurter Algemeine Zeitung* reporter if he had observed any new symptoms, Dr Streeck replied that 'a good two-thirds' described a loss of smell and taste over several days.

This goes so far that a mother could not smell the smell of a full diaper on her child. Others couldn't smell their shampoo any more, and food was beginning to taste bland. We cannot yet say exactly when these symptoms will occur, but we believe it will be a little later in the infection. The typical Covid-19 patient shows only mild symptoms.

Sudden onset anosmia was, for the first time, on the public record in Europe – if only in one newspaper – as a possible Covid symptom. Dr Streeck, however, was not the only physician that made the connection. In the Jiaotong University Health Science Centre in Xi'an, China, Dr Jingguo Chen, an ENT specialist, had read a report of a Chinese patient who had experienced smell loss as a first symptom of Covid back in February. He immediately embarked on a deep dive into the research literature and identified a female patient who had experienced anosmia after infection with SARS in 2006 in Taiwan. Trusting his instincts alone, he wrote an article for Chinese media published in the middle of March 2020, hoping to raise awareness of the possibility of a connection between olfactory dysfunction and Covid.

Growing patient anxieties saw Dr Jimmy Kyaw Tun, a consultant radiologist at St Bartholomew's Hospital in London's Smithfield, go public. He used Twitter to announce he would self-isolate despite the NHS's refusal to accept that his smell loss could be related and test him for Covid. Replies came back thick and fast from UK Twitter users who asked why Public Health England wasn't updating its guidelines to order self-isolation.

In the United States, patients were feeling similar frustrations. 'HollyA' from Seattle thanked the others for simply tweeting their experiences: 'This thread made me feel sane, thank you.' On the video-sharing social media site TikTok, newly anosmic patients filmed themselves chewing chillies and eating whole onions and lemons to illustrate the devastating extent of their smell loss. Social media influencers with large followings also chimed in, among them US actress Rachel Matthews, known for her voice-over in the film *Frozen 2*. She had reported on 17 March via her Instagram account that she had 'randomly lost my sense of smell and taste' on the fourth day after falling ill. The NBA star Rudy Gobert-Bourgarel was not far behind: 'Just to give you guys an update, loss of smell and taste is definitely one of the symptoms. Haven't been able to smell anything for the last four days.'

On 24 March, in South Korea, the Daegu City Medical Association also announced that it had conducted a telephone monitoring survey of 3,192 residents who had tested positive for Covid. Explaining the results to news agency, JoongAng Ilbo, doctors said that of the total, 488 who reported a fever or sore throat also stated they had lost their sense of smell and taste. However, when the 1,462 who had described themselves as asymptomatic were questioned a second time, a further 451 revealed disruption to their sense of smell and taste.

Evidence was mounting.

❖

Back in Umbria, despite his own growing suspicions, Dr Dehgani-Mobaraki was still at work, working seven days straight and sleeping in the hospital. His fiancée had also become sick. Without fever or cough, his anosmia did not fit the protocol for a Covid test and he was ordered to remain at work. Suspicious and anxious, he chose to work in full PPE including respirator mask, despite the hazmat look alarming his patients. 'I could not get off my job,' he recalled. 'At the time nobody was allowed to stay home and everyone was needed and was working every single day.'

It would be another eight days after he first sounded the alarm – and only when the young doctor reported feeling dizzy and his oxygen saturation levels suddenly dropped – that a PCR test was performed. Dr Dehgani-Mobaraki's results confirmed he was Covid positive. He was finally allowed to quarantine and spent the next forty days fighting the virus himself.

10

Science on the Scent

Claire Hopkins, Professor of Rhinology at Guy's and
St Thomas' Hospital in London, was already perplexed
about what she was hearing on the grapevine when Dr Dehgani-
Mobaraki's email from Italy pinged into her inbox. A specialist
in nasal and sinus disorders, particularly nasal polyps, Professor
Hopkins was used to seeing the occasional patient who presented
complaining about losing their sense of smell. Anosmia can strike
in the wake of a cold or flu when mucus, congestion and inflammation bungs up the airways, preventing smell molecules from
reaching the receptors. Hopkins estimated she'd seen at most one
anosmic patient a month in previous years – but now she'd seen
several in the preceding week. 'In my clinic the following Monday,
16 March, I saw four healthy young patients that had suddenly
lost their sense of smell but had no other symptoms at all,' she
recounted. 'One had flown back from San Francisco some weeks
earlier. Importantly they had no rhinitis, no cough, no fever.'

Hopkins' first instinct had been that the symptom was related
to post-viral loss, which is seasonal and often increases in March.
However, the absence of other symptoms was undoubtedly

odd and so she decided to dig around and look for any other real-time data that might link it to the new virus. That very afternoon, another email arrived, this one from medical colleagues in Treviso, in northern Italy. They also reported seeing a flurry of patients presenting with a loss of smell and asked if she could help evaluate them. By then, Hopkins had found and read German newspaper reports of data provided by her colleague Hendrik Streeck suggesting that as many as two in three Covid patients had lost their sense of smell as well as the earlier report from South Korea. Neither of these clarified whether patients had the more classic symptoms of Covid of cough and fever or whether smell loss was their only symptom.

Unable to find anything helpful in English-language media, medical literature or on the internet, Hopkins kept her growing suspicions to herself until she noticed a discussion on the rhinological section of the medical collaboration platform, DocMatter. A French ENT specialist, Ali Abbas, posted that he too was seeing more and more Covid patients but the critical point for Hopkins was that he reported they were presenting without any other symptoms, just a sudden loss of smell. The following day, another four patients arrived in her clinic, all complaining of the same thing. Hopkins had no way of checking the medical veracity of her intuition because only patients who had returned from Italy, Iran or China with a cough or fever were eligible for Covid testing. What is more, Public Health England was still advising that there was no significant risk of community-acquired Covid outside this group of returning travellers. What should she do?

Then she learned that a British ENT colleague, Amged El-Hawrani, an associate clinical director at University Hospitals of Derby and Burton, had been admitted to intensive care suffering Covid symptoms. (Aged just fifty-five, he would die on 28 March, the first UK doctor to become a casualty of the coronavirus.) For Professor Hopkins, El-Hawrani's hospitalisation was the impetus for action but, sensitive to the risks of raising a false alarm, she decided to write directly to Public Health England to voice her concerns. She told me:

> I realised that examining the nose of an infected patient with an endoscope or directly without PPE was potentially a very high-risk procedure due both to close contact and the risk of triggering a sneeze or cough while directly in front of the patient. I also realised that there was a significant public-health benefit in reducing transmission if this was a way to identify otherwise asymptomatic patients who were otherwise well enough to carry on with normal activities.

On 19 March, she felt it necessary to contact her colleague Professor Nirmal Kumar, President of ENT UK, to ask if he would join her in countersigning a warning letter to their members advising caution and urging the use of PPE when seeing patients with sudden loss of smell. He agreed:

> We also recommended that anyone with sudden loss of smell should isolate . . . there are very few causes for sudden loss of smell in young healthy people other than post-viral and in the absence of head trauma and the risk of harm seemed to be low and greatly outweighed by the potential benefits.

The following day, six days after Dr Mobaraki's anxious email, Professor Hopkins and Professor Kumar took the unprecedented decision to publish their own public warning on Twitter as well, urging recognition of loss of smell as an early marker of Covid infection and urging the need for self-isolation. The tweet was shared nearly 4,000 times but in the UK at least fell on deaf ears. The letter was the first English-language report to warn of anosmia as a symptom of Covid and was rapidly picked up by news media worldwide.

Hopkins quickly turned to work on the data collected by her Italian colleague, Paolo Boscolo-Rizzo, and the team in Treviso. Their paper was accepted for publication by *JAMA*, the American Medical Association's open access network just ten days later. The battle to have anosmia recognised as a symptom of Covid, however, had only just begun.

❖

A couple of days before Puppysnot sent her anguished question into cyberspace, Dr Maria Veldhuizen, a research scientist with the Department of Anatomy at Mersin University in Turkey, had been at her laptop working remotely when she too began to take notice of a growing flurry of unconfirmed reports of sudden-onset anosmia. She recalls them as no more than 'murmurs' from Iran, Italy and Israel but, true to her discipline, her curiosity was sparked immediately and she started to think about ways to test their veracity in a safe but scientifically rigorous way. On 19 March, the same day Professor Claire Hopkins issued her warning, Dr Veldhuizen typed the hashtag #Covid19 into her Twitter account and, on a whim, asked if any colleagues knew of home taste/smell tests using household items that might be used with patients. 'Not for diagnostic purposes', she wrote, 'but to track olfactory function during an epidemic.' Adding the hashtag #citizen-science, she asked 'for an RT' and posted.

It took less than seventy-two hours for her appeal to reverberate globally. Clinicians, neuroscientists, psychology researchers, philosophers, biologists and chemists from the UK, Netherlands, Florida and Pennsylvania in the US, Denmark, Sweden, Germany and Italy not only retweeted but joined the conversation, bandying about ideas on how to collaborate and test if it really was the new virus wreaking such a seemingly devastating effect on the olfactory system.

Every day that she logged on, more people seemed keen to enter the discussion: Ilja Croijmans, an olfaction researcher in Utrecht, offered up his undergraduate students to help out: 'They can't do their planned lab experiments any more.' Professor Barry Smith in London suggested a test to clarify quickly if it was smell, not taste, that had been affected: 'Home testing . . . is easy to set up. Placing salt, sugar or lemon juice on the tongue. Asking if people can smell/feel the tingle in mint, can feel the burning sensation of mustard. Does toothpaste still tingle? Sniff soaps.'

On 24 March, the nascent group held a first virtual meeting and the following day, a German chemosensory researcher Kathrin Ohla tweeted ecstatically: 'Have you ever wondered whether you can hold a structured and productive video call with 75 participants? You can. We did. #Chemosensory enthusiasts rock!'

Four days later, the group had grown to 100 and they decided on a name for their pioneering open-science project: the Global

Consortium for Chemosensory Research – GCCR for short – was born. It was decided quickly that discussions needed to be moved from Twitter to a more manageable but equally democratic platform and a leadership team was nominated to take on specific tasks.

Valentina Parma, a young Italian neuroscientist working as Research Assistant Professor in Psychology at Temple University in Philadelphia, was thrust into the chair's role. 'I'm not very good on Twitter so I was looped in a little later and asked to jump on a call,' she told me with a smile, her newborn baby cooing in the background. 'They said to me, "C'mon, you know how to get people organised, you can chair." It happened just like that.' Slack, pretty much a messaging service on steroids, offered its services free to the scientists and, buoyed by the ability to converse so easily, they began work, forgetting language and time differences.

At the heart of the debate lay the need to find a way to harness mass patient experience in the most scientifically credible manner. Did they want to conduct a series of short surveys or one, long, detailed patient questionnaire? How best could they do this? As researchers, they recognised the opportunity presented by the global phenomenon of mass anosmia but while patients were not being tested for Covid the symptom remained anecdotal. It was clear that time was of the essence and while some voiced understandable doubts about how best to deal with the situation, others feared the loss of valuable information if they didn't seize the moment.

Dresden University's Professor Thomas Hummel, one of the world's leading olfactory researchers, immediately stepped in to provide the group with patient and clinical perspective. Professor Steven Munger, director of the Centre for Smell and Taste at the University of Florida, offered his considerable experience as chair of another large scientific organisation. The geneticist Danielle Reed from the Monell Chemical Senses Center in Pennsylvania – known in the olfactory world for identifying the receptors that detect bitter flavours – was able to draw on her connections with other research consortia. In the UK, Chrissi Kelly offered her burgeoning patient advocacy experience with AbScent. The group had quickly concluded that the best way to gather data was to appeal directly to sufferers and began work on constructing a detailed questionnaire designed to elicit the information researchers desperately needed to answer their questions.

Issues of inclusivity, language translation, data science and ethics were thrashed out into the early hours and Pennsylvania State University's Professor John Hayes stepped in to help steer the Institutional Review Board approval that is always needed when research involves human subjects. It was not all roses: some researchers felt speed was of the essence and new research models needed to be found that might require bypassing the usual protocols for research while many others were sticklers for the traditional pre-publication hurdles that would slow the pace. Frustrations bubbled but all agreed that smell – the neglected sense – and anosmia – the invisible problem unrecognised as important by so many GPs – was suddenly in the public spotlight. A tweet sent by Chrissi Kelly encapsulated the sense of opportunity and excitement felt in the relatively small world of global olfactory research: 'It is impossible to see a silver lining anywhere in a global health emergency like the one we are in now. But smell, has at last been pushed to the forefront. What new avenues will be discovered in our research?'

※

As the GCCR continued to grow – to 500 by the end of March – it attracted an even wider array of members interested in smell: food scientists and nutritionists, perfumers and sommeliers, microbiologists and geneticists, artists and writers. The various members were taken aback at the extraordinary range of disciplines and interests the group represented. Dr Anna-Lisa D'Errico, a neuroscientist with a passion for the use of odours in theatre, exemplified the eclectic and complex interplay of minds at work in the GCCR. The author of an Italian-language book on the nose and sense of smell, she told me she was driven to join GCCR early by the desire to collaborate and communicate at a time when Italians were desperate for information. 'I just wanted to help fill the gap between science and the general public.' She was also quick to remind me that the olfactory sciences are still young: 'We still don't know how the communication between the olfactory bulb and cortex works. It's puzzling and, while we have learned a lot, there is still so much that is unclear.'

Clinical studies for publication and peer review often take several months or longer to develop, but as Covid threatened to envelop the world at a terrifying pace, the group vowed to set aside personal academic or professional progress to work collaboratively and ensure similar speeds.

Their mission would receive a significant scientific fillip: Harvard Medical Schools' Professor of Neurology, Sandeep Robert Datta, pre-published a ground-breaking paper,[1] which confirmed not only that the Covid virus attacked the nose but exactly where it wreaked damage.

The members of Datta's team had initially thrown themselves into exploring the relationship between anosmia and the virus by examining the olfactory genes, but in early March laboratories began to understand the implications of the virus and prepared to close. 'To tell a team to stop and go home was awful,' he told me, sipping a coffee one summer morning.

A member of the GCCR himself, Datta started to look around to see what might be explored outside an experimental setting: 'We put our heads together on what data we might already have in the can or what data our friends might have to shed light on what was happening.'

Datta and his team decided to turn first to publicly available genetics data to look at how the virus might be entering the olfactory system before going on to disrupt its function. He soon realised that his lab had already conducted a series of experiments to try to identify which specific genes are expressed by which specific cells in the nose and decided to return to these results to see if they offered any insights into how the virus might attack the sense of smell. (Gene expression is the process by which information stored in DNA is converted into instructions for making specialised proteins or other molecules.)

They focused first on the olfactory epithelium and the two proteins that had already been identified as receptors of the coronavirus. Chinese scientists had unmasked the viral genome with inordinate speed and published it in January while the spike proteins that help the virus to lock onto the surface of human cells via the receptor known as ACE-2 had been identified a month later. Datta's instinct told him that the cells that expressed these molecules in the epithelium could well make them uniquely susceptible to attack by Covid. But when the researchers got down to testing the theory, trawling through the data to see if the cells contained ACE-2 and the other protein that helps SARS-CoV-2 get into our cells, they got a huge surprise. It wasn't the sensory neurones themselves but the supporting cells around them that had succumbed to Covid. Known as sustentacular cells, these act just like scaffolding around a building, helping keep the complex neuronal structures in place:

> We were working from home and when we got the first in silico results [experiments performed by computer], we were pretty bowled over because we pretty much expected that the virus, given its profound and sudden effect on the sense of smell, would attack the cells responsible for conveying information about odorants from your nose to the brain. When we saw that wasn't the case, we knew it could be a potentially important result because it might explain the other weird thing about Covid anosmia, which is that people were losing it suddenly, like a light switch, and while some were getting it back quite quickly, with others the loss was more persistent. The model that the virus just attacked the sensory neurones willy-nilly just didn't accommodate these two kinds of patients.

Clinicians knew that if the neurones had been the centre of damage, the likelihood is that all patients would lose their sense of smell for a very long time. Datta noted:

You have to rebuild the whole system and that would take forever. Most patients lose it for some weeks but then get it back while others are still doing really badly . . . that is a thing we had never seen before. So, infection of the sustentacular cells explained both modes of the disease.

Datta says the group's find highlighted just how little was known about this part of our nasal system:

We consider ourselves experts in the basic functions of the olfactory system and yet we had never considered them until then. There is so much more science to be done.

At last, here was data-driven, laboratory evidence of a link between Covid and sudden onset anosmia.

Many months later, another American multi-university team, which was working with golden hamsters infected with Covid, confirmed that the virus does not invade the neurones themselves but the scaffolding cells that hold them up and it is the resulting inflammation – the immune system's 'friendly fire' – that sends smell AWOL.[2]

But would the GCCR manage to set aside the natural, scientific bent towards process and manage to disseminate their questionnaire and crunch the numbers in time to make a real difference?

11

In AbScentia

Anosmia Awareness Day had been celebrated on 27 February, just three weeks before doctors around the world began to report sudden-onset smell loss in Covid patients. The brainchild of an American man with congenital anosmia, Daniel Schein, it had begun as a small event, on Facebook in 2012, garnering more support over the years as new charities and research institutions spread awareness of the little-known syndrome.

In the UK, Chrissi Kelly had been preparing for the 2020 event oblivious to what was about to explode around her. 'I'd had this idea to send AbScent key lanyards out to all the olfactory scientists, clinicians and research groups we'd worked with over the years to say thank you,' she recalled. AbScent had about 1,500 members on its Facebook page on Anosmia Day but they had more than doubled a week later and would grow exponentially as each day passed. Within a fortnight, the original anosmia group had been swamped and Kelly, who had started her group in 2015, knew something very, very strange was happening.

She was only too aware that those who had suffered anosmia without attention for years were, in her own words, 'getting hacked off' by the new circumstances. So she decided it was time to create a separate Covid anosmia page for the newbies. At 10.30 p.m. on 24 March, after a long and tiring day, she pulled an image of a generic, luminous green virus from the internet, stuck it on the top of a new Facebook page with the title 'Covid-19 Smell and Taste Loss', pressed the button to launch and retired to bed. When she got up less than eight hours later, 650 new people had joined, all sharing their anxiety and bewilderment at the sudden loss of their fifth sense.

Shocked, Kelly realised that this was also the day the new scientific group, GCCR, was to hold its first virtual meeting. Later she told me:

When I joined them, I said, 'If you want your own Petri dish, here it is. I'm offering you 650 new people and that's just from the last few hours. It felt a little like when you drop an egg into swirling water to poach. Suddenly it coalesces, it comes together and we found ourselves with this incredible number of patients who were talking about what was happening to them in real time. I just happened to find myself at the epicentre of it all.

I discovered Chrissi Kelly and AbScent's Covid anosmia page a few days after my own sense of smell had disappeared. For me, as an expatriate Italian Australian living in the UK, Facebook has long been a lifeline to keep in contact with friends and family in both countries as well as a sort of stand-in for the watercooler discussions about breaking news I used to love sharing with journalistic colleagues at my old newspaper. My memory of that afternoon – 27 March – when the anosmia took hold is etched indelibly and I see my movements in slow motion, the feeling of unreality and utter disconnection intermingled with a sinking sensation of doom. Somehow, it felt instinctive to key in 'loss of smell' on Facebook itself and AbScent's bright-green Covid page popped up instantly. Within minutes I read of scores of people as mystified and as desperate as me who had shared their tales: 'It was like a light switch from 100 per cent to zero per cent in a couple of hours . . . it's like my nose is switched off,' posted one. 'My taste and smell left on Sunday, very suddenly. One minute I was eating, the next it had gone', and yet another, 'You feel so detached from reality when you can't smell your surroundings.'

I would learn too that another group of doctors halfway around the world in Iran published their work that same day, this time using information collected from 10,069 patients seen between 12 and 17 March in Tehran.[1] Led by the University of Medical Sciences' Seyed Hamidreza Bagheri, they found that 'sudden-onset anosmia was seen in over 76 per cent of cases'. The paper was uploaded onto the pre-publication site, medRxiv, with remarkable speed, adding further real-time data to the growing, global argument for recognition of anosmia as a Covid symptom.

The clamour for self-isolation and special precautions was growing but was still being met with a resounding silence from health authorities.

◆

Good science is often about the long, hard slog. And yet some of the greatest discoveries throughout history are also serendipitous.

Alexander Fleming's discovery of penicillin while researching the influenza virus in 1928 is a great example. He had been working in the laboratory at St Mary's Hospital in London when he returned from a two-week holiday only to find that a careless lab technician had allowed the contamination of a staphylococcus culture plate with mould. When Fleming examined the mould, he realised immediately that it appeared to have prevented the growth of the bacteria. That freak moment changed our health and the modern medical world. (A more recent and amusing chance find must be Pfizer's development of Viagra: the blue pill began life as a new treatment for angina but turned out to be useless – until researchers started to hear reports of its other, unexpected side-effect.)

As the GCCR grew even more, its members representing nearly fifty nations, work slowed, perhaps stymied a little by size, politics and logistics, while serendipity struck a smaller and perhaps more nimble outfit at King's College London. Tim Spector, a professor of genetic epidemiology, had spent eighteen years studying twins after founding the UK's largest twins registry, TwinsUK, in 1992. His interest lay in working out how two people with identical genes could grow up to develop completely different diseases, as well as characteristics. Spector focused on nutrition among other areas, looking at how they might share the same diet but develop different allergies or have metabolisms that responded differently to similar blood sugar levels.

In 2018, a year before Covid emerged in China, Spector had joined forces with two tech specialists, Jonathan Wolf and George Hadjigeorgiou, to create ZOE, a commercial start-up that aimed, rather ambitiously, to build the largest nutrition study in the world. Their business plan was to use machine learning to utilise the enormous amount of data on the impact of genes, life-style and gut bacteria (microbiome) gathered by Spector's work to develop a personalised app to help consumers make the best food choices based on physiology. Work had begun with twins pretty much straight away and quickly expanded into a partnership with another research institution in Boston in the United States.

And then Covid happened.

On 20 March, as the new virus began to envelop the world, Spector took the prescient decision to turn to his TwinsUK volunteers and try to track the symptoms and trajectory of the virus. Serendipitously, he hauled in his ZOE colleagues to tweak the app to help the twins and test volunteers to log their symptoms. (This aspect proved impossible in the early days until the UK testing regime became more widespread.)

Hadjigeorgiou and his team realised very quickly that the app could be used much more widely, perhaps even to gauge how the virus was progressing through the UK as well as to crunch the reams of incoming demographic and geographic data. The members of the group – perhaps with an eye on a potential future contract with the NHS – put together what they described as a 'SWAT team' and by the end of that weekend, the ZOE Covid symptom tracker was born. The app went live on 24 March and by the following day, fuelled by burgeoning Covid case numbers, more than a million people had downloaded it.

It seems incredible in hindsight but in less than a week, the ZOE team was able to analyse symptom reports from 400,000 people: the sudden loss of smell and taste was proving to be a common sign of coronavirus infection: nearly one in five had reported the symptom.

Press reports of the ZOE group's first data crunch showed that 53 per cent of the 400,000 respondents had experienced fatigue, 29 per cent a cough, 28 per cent shortness of breath and 18 per cent loss of smell. Just 10.5 per cent reported fever. Even though the level of testing was very low, with less than 600 reported cases, of these almost two-thirds had reported a loss of smell.[2]

Spector and his team, mindful of NHS and government reticence on the issue and perhaps reluctant to seem to be contradicting official advice, stated clearly in their public statement that loss of smell and taste *might* be useful extra symptoms. However, they too were convinced enough to advocate being safe rather than sorry, adding strength to the earlier warning issued by Claire Hopkins and her colleagues. Spector said, 'When combined with other symptoms, people with loss of smell and taste appear to be three times more likely to have contracted Covid-19 according to our data, and should therefore self- isolate for seven days to reduce the spread of the disease.'

Three senior and experienced clinicians – Claire Hopkins, Nirmal Kumar, then Spector with the ZOE app – had made their beliefs very clear. Not long after, they were joined by the World Health Organization in Geneva. In the UK, however, anosmia was not yet recognised as a symptom of Covid.

●

For Kelly, the clamour from patients was starting to become overwhelming. As the days passed and health systems in the UK, the US and Europe recorded the exponential growth in positive cases, so too did the AbScent anosmia Facebook group. Applications for membership came not just from the English-speaking world but from Brazil, Italy, India, Spain and France. Kelly, whose personal experience of long-haul anosmia gave her a powerful empathy for those finding themselves newly lacking the fifth sense, found herself working fourteen-hour days as she tried to respond and reassure the tsunami of distressed and desperate people. She moderated the page herself, vetting each application to join it and trying to ensure that posts related solely to the issue and that any information provided was fact-checked and evidence-based. Kelly remembers beginning to notice geographic patterns as a flurry of respondents would come from a particular region of the UK or Europe followed by reports of infection spikes.

Her role appeared to be a textbook case of the phenomenon described by Professor Arthur Frank, now emeritus professor of sociology at the University of Calgary, in his seminal 1993 book *The Wounded Storyteller*. Republished several times since, it tells the story of his own cancer diagnosis, chronicling what it is like living with illness in the era of modern medicine. Frank describes the growing cohort of people who survive previously killer diseases as the 'remission society', arguing that patients often pass through a 'chaos and quest narrative' as they try to carve out a decent way to live with chronic sickness or disability. Chaos erupts as they and their loved ones try to process and make sense of the diagnosis while the 'quest' part of the journey is about finding others with similar stories to help push out the sense of isolation and find solace in shared experience.

This is exactly what the Facebook group, fast approaching 10,000 members, appeared to be doing. Kelly told me:

Just learning a little about the sense of smell, how it works and finding a language and words helped people makes sense of what was going on for them. Even knowing there is a word for it, a medical term – anosmia – gave them something to hang on to. So many people posted about how hard it was to explain to family members or even for their experience to be believed. Sharing what was happening to them helped both to normalise and also to reassure.

I know how panicked I felt in the early days of anosmia and yet I was one of the lucky ones, able to access fresh information as it became available while reporting the pandemic as well as tapping into what clinicians, including my ICU-specialist brother, Richard, in Australia, could share with me. Patients posting on the AbScent page from both sides of the Atlantic were less fortunate and railed daily against clinicians who dismissed their questions or simply told them to return in a few months without offering an explanation let alone a prognosis. Many reported being infuriated or deeply hurt when told they should be grateful that they'd not had severe or life-threatening symptoms and had 'only' lost their sense of smell. All reported the distress and strangeness of being guinea pigs with a little-understood dysfunction and the debilitating effects of 'feeling like it will be years' before medical knowledge would be able to catch up with what was happening to them.

12

A Political Stink

The day 3 April 2020 was one of the darkest for the UK, the deadliest since the beginning of the pandemic. Prime Minister Boris Johnson was the first world leader to succumb to the virus and despite attempts by his office to convince the public that he had only mild symptoms, he was about to be hospitalised and have a brush with death. His Health Secretary, Matt Hancock, had only just returned to work himself, forced to isolate at home for more than a week after testing positive for Covid. Hancock spent the first morning back on a media blitz, insisting the PM was fine while offering a rather more frank view of his own Covid experience: a throat so sore it felt as if it were filled with glass shards, rapid weight loss and the psychological struggle with anxiety about how his lungs might fare. During the interviews he revealed another experience – the sudden loss of the sense of taste. What in retrospect was anosmia and ageusia, once again, went unremarked by journalists.

That night, Hancock also fronted the televised Downing Street media briefing that would quickly become compulsive viewing as millions of households across the nation settled nervously into the second week of a three-month lockdown. By now, almost 3,500 people had died and hospitalisations were rising rapidly as case numbers, hidden behind a woefully low testing regime, exploded across the country. Standing beside Hancock that evening were Deputy Chief Medical Officer (DCMO) Dr Jonathan Van-Tam and Chief Nursing Officer Ruth May.

When the time came for questions, Robert Peston, political editor of ITV, raised the question of loss of taste and smell, asking if it would be added to the official list of symptoms: 'Are you looking at changing the guidelines to people for when they quarantine, because at the moment you're saying self-isolate if it's a high fever and a cough, but are you going to add to the list of symptoms where people should start self-isolating?'

It wasn't the first time the issue had been raised.

Just four days earlier, the government's chief scientific adviser, Sir Patrick Vallance, had offered his opinion that loss of taste and smell 'does seem to be a feature of this, from what people are reporting, and it is obviously something that people should take into account as they think about their symptoms'. Hancock's response seemed to confirm his adviser's view. After thanking Peston for the scientific questions and joking he intended passing the buck straight to Van-Tam, Hancock offered a personal answer to the query about anosmia: 'I did lose my sense of taste and that actually has begun to come back though. I can assure people who have lost their sense of taste that the good news is that, in my case, it wasn't permanent.'

Van-Tam frowned over the reading glasses perched on the end of his nose, and made clear his contrary view:

We have actually asked our expert advisory committee NERVTAG [New and Emerging Virus Threats Advisory Group] to look at this. There are some anecdotal data that are now in the published domain that suggests that a proportion of people do indeed lose their sense of taste and smell. However, we have looked at the data in relation to whether it is a symptom that would be important to add to the case definition. The answer from our experts is absolutely not. As far as we can tell on limited data it doesn't contribute anything on its own to the overall affinity of the diagnosis.

Not only had the DCMO refused to accept the warnings of olfactory scientists and clinicians, but he had taken the inexplicable step of categorically ruling anosmia out as a symptom. It was a devastating moment, confirmed by media headlines that night and into the next morning which all repeated Van-Tam's exact words: Anosmia would 'absolutely not' be added to the list of symptoms.

ENT UK chief, Professor Nirmal Kumar, expressed his disappointment immediately and publicly, adding that not only would he continue to tell his own patients to self-isolate but would also encourage people to 'sniff out Covid', regularly testing their sense of smell with household items such as coffee to rule out unexplained anosmia.

Behind the scenes, Professor Claire Hopkins, her ENT colleague Simon Gane, Professor Barry Smith and Chrissi Kelly among others were 'tearing their hair out'. Barry Smith recalled:

We were hearing from people in ICUs and the medical front line that they were calling 111 to report anosmia and being told they didn't have Covid. We were now in a Catch-22: we knew this was a symptom but you couldn't be tested unless you were symptomatic but loss of smell wasn't a symptom and so you couldn't get a test and so it went, around and around.

Van-Tam's outright dismissal appeared even more incongruous in the light of what had unfolded internally, behind the scenes. Professor Peter Rea, a consultant ENT surgeon in Leicester, and Claire Hopkins had also sent an email to several Public Health England contacts asking it be passed onto senior officials:

> The President of the British Rhinology Society in collaboration with colleagues in Italy and Iran have identified a potentially important marker of occult Covid-19 infection. They are seeing large numbers of infected patients presenting with anosmia only and no other symptoms. They may be a large pool of unwitting super-spreaders. They believe by instructing the population who lose their sense of smell to self-isolate the spread of infection may be slowed.

Hopkins followed up on her warning during a meeting with officials from PHE's TARGET division, known by its acronym due to its mind-boggling long title – the Tuberculosis, Acute Respiratory, Gastrointestinal, Emerging/zoonotic Infections and Travel arm. During discussions, officials agreed to add questions about the loss of smell to their own ongoing research on the first

1,000 patients testing positive for Covid. They also suggested to Hopkins that she make contact with Tim Spector and ask that his team add a question about loss of smell and taste to the ZOE symptom-tracker app. Hopkins' written request would be the catalyst for the ZOE team's push to gather data to demonstrate the significance of smell loss.

This was not the only work: further studies had been set in train by scientists at the Defence Science and Technology Laboratory (DSTL). Effectively the scientific arm of the UK Ministry of Defence, research teams there had been deployed to conduct several studies aimed at identifying the behaviour and viability of the Covid virus in aerosol droplets and in enclosed environments. This would be hugely important information for clinicians making policy on how to manage so-called asymptomatic, anosmic carriers.

Copies of NERVTAG meeting minutes also showed that anosmia had been raised in that forum too, the first time during a video-link meeting on 27 March when members had been presented with what was described as 'soft intelligence' from France and Italy. The loss of smell and taste returned to the agenda one week later – the day of the Hancock press conference – with the minutes recording a summary by NERVTAG chairman, Professor Peter Horby, director of Oxford University's epidemic diseases research group, who stated that 'anosmia/ageusia were credible symptoms for consideration in clinical case definitions'. The minutes show he added a caveat that 'more data are required before consideration is given to changing the case definition'.

To be fair, the UK was not alone in hesitating to accept the loss of smell and taste as a symptom. However, as the days went by, evidence reported by patients around the world kept mounting exponentially. On 1 April the GCCR had made public the preliminary findings of its global, multi-language survey of more than 4,000 patients.[1] This concluded that smell, taste and chemesthesis – perception of irritants such as chilli and wasabi – drop significantly in patients testing positive for Covid and that this decline in senses was the 'best predictor of infection'. *Nature* magazine also reported updated ZOE figures, derived not only from the now 2.5 million contributors in the UK but also a growing cohort of app users in the United States. The survey concluded that 65 per cent of the 7,000 respondents who had tested positive for Covid reported a loss of taste and smell. Given the continued lack of available testing in the UK and the US, the authors reported, it was becoming even more important to include anosmia as indicative of a need for immediate self-isolation.

France would be the first country to take decisive action and at the daily, national televised briefing on 23 March the director-general of the French health service, Jérôme Salomon, delivered an unequivocal message: 'If you suffer from a sudden loss of taste or smell, you are advised to call your doctor.' Germany, under the assured leadership of Angela Merkel, a former research scientist with a doctorate in quantum chemistry, was more hesitant but by the middle of April its national public health body, the Robert Koch Institute, was issuing comprehensive daily updates including loss of smell or taste as a symptom suggesting that at least 15 per cent of new cases reported the loss of one or both.

Even the United States, fractured by disparate state responses to the pandemic and the increasingly bizarre behaviour of President Donald Trump, moved to add anosmia to the symptom list. On 17 April the US Centers for Disease Control and Prevention (CDC), under pressure from the American Academy of Otolaryngology (the study of the ear and throat) – which had launched its own anosmia reporting tool – formally added anosmia to its symptoms list. The World Health Organization (WHO) followed suit the same day, prompting a further rash of changes around the world, including a European Union decree.

Back in London, they were still dithering. NERVTAG had scheduled a meeting on the same day as the WHO and CDC announcements and the minutes show that members discussed the results of yet another study, this one from the United States noting that 60 per cent of positive cases had reported anosmia. 'There appears to be a consistent signal that anosmia may occur in Covid-19 infection,' the NERVTAG minutes concluded. 'An answer on whether anosmia should be included in the case definition will be an important policy question going forward.'

A further two weeks would pass before the issue was raised again, this time in relation to the contact-tracing app being developed by the NHS. There was now an urgent need to finalise the set of symptoms to be included on the app when it was launched. The action plan from the meeting of 1 May noted: 'NERVTAG and DCMO [Jonathan Van-Tam] to finalise assessment of anosmia and consider other symptom clusters which might be critical to rapid contact tracing.'

This 'consensus view' was sent on Sunday 3 May to the Department of Health and Social Care, headed by the Chief Medical Officer, Chris Whitty, and his Deputy, Jonathan Van-Tam.

The decision would be delayed yet again. Insiders recalled that NERVTAG's next meeting ran over, forcing postponement of discussion of the new evidence while an early May Bank Holiday weekend postponed consideration again. Every hour is important when an infectious, airborne respiratory virus is at play and by this stage many in Britain's medical and scientific community were both panicked and infuriated. 'It was hard to see the rationale of why they were delaying,' Barry Smith recalled. 'The only reason we could see was that they simply didn't have the testing capacity to cope with an upsurge in demand if anosmia was formally noted as a symptom.' The other possibility was impact on the NHS: 'It was like the Greek tragedy of *Oedipus* . . . in the desire to avoid extra pressure on the NHS by denying anosmia, the government just created the conditions that would do exactly that.'

On 9 May, a frustrated Tim Spector hit the airwaves. Seventeen countries had now updated their advice to include anosmia and, as an epidemiologist, he could not understand why there was a continuing delay in the UK: 'Someone has got to urgently ask this question of why we're the only country in this crisis that isn't really widening our group of symptoms and get on with it and do something.'

Claire Hopkins took up the cudgels on the BBC on 12 May. The government, she said, could no longer deny what was by now 'robust' evidence:

We've been able to show that in groups of patients that have lost their sense of smell without any other symptoms, there's a greater than 95 per cent chance it is due to Covid-19. By contrast, fever is not a good marker because many things can cause a fever, and this symptom is only present in about 40 per cent of patients with Covid-19.

Behind the scenes, Barry Smith and his colleagues had also been quietly updating a senior BBC editor about the mounting evidence. Sceptical at first, the public broadcaster decided it was now time to explore the ramifications of delays if anosmia was not quickly added to the symptom list. Among the interviewees was a respiratory physiotherapist in the West Midlands who worked with cardio-pulmonary patients, possibly the most vulnerable patient cohort of all. He lost his sense of taste and smell but was told by the NHS Helpline that this was not a problem and to return to work. He ignored advice and self-isolated, as did his mother, a podiatrist working with elderly people and his sister, an intensive-care nurse. His boss ordered a test for him despite the protocols and it came back positive. 'Based on government advice alone, I would have been back at work, going from patient to patient and potentially giving them coronavirus,' he told the BBC.

And yet NERVTAG was still inexplicably hesitant. Asked to comment by the BBC, one member, Dr Ben Killingley, a consultant at UCL, and its chair, Professor Peter Horby, raised worries about 'false-positives'. During private discussions, NERVTAG moved to try to test anosmia as a symptom in a track-and-trace trial on the Isle of Wight.

On 18 May, Spector was back on the BBC's *Today* programme, warning that thousands of cases were being missed:

At the moment, people are being told to go back to work if they're a care worker, and they've got something like loss of

smell or taste or severe muscle pains or fatigue – things that
we know, and we've shown are related to being swabbed positive. This country is missing the ball in underestimated cases,
but also putting people at risk, and continuing the epidemic.

That night First Secretary of State Dominic Raab fronted the
Downing Street briefing. The situation was grim, he said. Deaths
across the United Kingdom were now almost 35,000, a tenfold
increase in the six weeks since 3 April. But, he insisted, there was
light at the end of the tunnel: the peak had been reached and
passed, helped by a surge in testing capacity, which had reached
100,000 or more each day while hospitalisations were slowly
decreasing. The worst appeared to be over, Raab told the press
conference, and the government would now launch its 'roadmap'
to guide the nation's release from lockdown while also preparing
for the possibility of a second wave: 'We are going to be very
mindful to avoid a second wave,' he pledged.

When the conference was thrown open to questions, the
BBC's medical editor, Fergus Walsh, raised the topic of anosmia: 'France advised people back in March that if they lost taste
or smell that they should self-isolate. Hasn't the UK been very
slow to act?'

Van-Tam's defence was strident. Although it was true that
anosmia had been recognised for some time as a possible symptom, it wasn't as simple as accepting there was a connection, he
insisted. Rather it had to be understood in terms of when in the
trajectory of the disease it appeared in comparison with coughs
and fever and how often it appeared as the only symptom, which,
he declared confidently, was 'very rarely indeed'.

The DCMO even appeared to dismiss the WHO's formal list of symptoms – 'tiredness, aches and pains, sore throat, diarrhoea, conjunctivitis, headache, skin rash, even loss of speech or movement' – as overly complicated, confusing and of little use in identifying patients:

> That's why we have taken our time in this country because we wanted to do that, again, painstaking and very careful analysis before we jumped to any conclusions. And even if it was barn-door-obvious that anosmia was part of this, we wanted to be sure that adding it to cough and fever, as opposed to just listing it, adding it in formally into our definition, was the right thing to do. And based on advice from NERVTAG, we have made that decision.

Fergus Walsh, a medical journalist, had a supplementary question up his sleeve:

> Tim Spector estimates that between 100,000 and 200,000 cases of Covid-19 may be missed by the failure to include this earlier. How many cases do you think have been missed as a result of not including this earlier on?

Van-Tam bristled. 'I'm not sure anyone other than Professor Spector is trying to make those kinds of estimates,' he shot back, insisting that Public Health England's own data, the so-called FF100 (first few hundred cases) study, recorded less than one per cent of patients having anosmia as the only symptom:

So the point about anosmia is that it doesn't always come as the first symptom. And even if it does, it is followed by the cough, the fever, and many of the other symptoms that I've talked about referring to the WHO definition. So you don't miss those cases. And the important thing was to work out if this would add any sensitivity to the diagnostic cluster we were using. And the answer is it makes a small, very small difference, and we have therefore decided to do it.

A few hours later, the UK's chief medical officers for England, Scotland, Wales and Northern Ireland went ahead and did what Claire Hopkins and the Italian physicians along with Barry Smith, Chrissi Kelly and countless others at the olfactory coalface had been saying for more than two months:

> From today, all individuals should self-isolate if they develop a new continuous cough or fever or anosmia. We have been closely monitoring the emerging data and evidence on Covid-19 and after thorough consideration, we are now confident enough to recommend this new measure. The individual's household should also self-isolate for fourteen days as per the current guidelines and the individual should stay at home for seven days, or longer if they still have symptoms other than cough or loss of sense of smell or taste.

It was a significant if pyrrhic victory because just as smell loss finally gained formal status as a Covid symptom, the virus threw out another curve ball as patients' noses began to return to life – and smell the unimaginable.

13

Smell Warp

One early morning during the brief summer break from lockdown, I woke up and went to the coffee machine, plonked the cup under the spout, pressed the button and went into the bathroom. By then, most smells were still barely perceptible but I was very aware they were returning and grateful they'd not distorted into the inferno described by so many others. I'd slowly taught myself to look for pleasures to compensate for flavour and enjoyed the familiar, wake-up ritual by focusing on the little rush of caffeine energy because, truthfully, if blindfolded, I'd not be able to discern an espresso from a cup of sweetened tea. However, that morning, when I grabbed the cup from the machine, I was unexpectedly swamped by a new and indescribable smell, one that bore no resemblance to the roasty, bitter-smoky scent of coffee as I once knew it although, thankfully, it didn't elicit disgust. Rather, it struck me as earthy-sweet, utterly dissonant, incongruous, wrong.

Baffled, I downed the shot anyway because, by then, I was becoming accustomed to the curveballs thrown by a malfunctioning fifth sense, simply adding such moments to my calendar as an aide-memoire. What happened next fell outside the perplexing and into the surreal: I went to the bathroom and the smell of poo (sorry, readers!), which until then had been entirely absent from my olfactory lexicon, was exactly like this 'new' coffee. Unlike those afflicted by textbook parosmia, I'd had the opposite and not smelled 'bathroom smells' for months: no teenage farts, no stinky loos, no dog poos – absolutely nothing. If I had a pound for every person who told me I should be happy about this, I'd be rich indeed. Still, they were right in a way; some people's experiences were far worse. Many months later I was to meet Cara Roberts, who had become anosmic through Covid in December 2020 and in March was struck by a bout of parosmia so ferocious that she ended up on intravenous anti-nausea medication in hospital after losing two stone in three weeks. However, so little was known of the condition then that she was placed on a ward for eating disorders. 'I thought I was going mad, nobody believed me,' she remembers. 'I heard a nurse at change of shift say: "She thinks her food doesn't taste right and makes herself sick." Nobody knew anything about it then. Even now, so many people who have shared their experiences with me via Instagram @parosmia_diaries say that many doctors and ENT specialists still don't know much about it. It's much better now and sharing experiences is so helpful.'

My nose's response recovery was indeed less extreme but it became one of the most unsettling aspects of anosmia because, whether we like it or not, we smell-test ourselves often to gauge the state of our body and its health. We may not be aware of it but we appear to be wired to perceive changes in faecal or urine smells, or if body odour or breath appears more sweet or acrid than usual. Perhaps modern humans do not always act on these stimuli but I realised then that it's something I must have monitored often, if unconsciously, and I felt strange without it.

I would learn that it is an area of new and fascinating research; an Israeli study, published in April 2020 just as the pandemic began to take hold, had examined the frequency with which humans touch their faces and found it to be similar to that observed in primates such as orangutans.[1] In a twenty-minute observation period, participants touched their faces an average of nearly fourteen times and researchers argued that this face-touching, while largely unconscious, is not only a form of subliminal, instinctive self-smelling but also a touchstone for where their hands had been previously. When asked about sniffing their own bodies or those of their familiars, 94 per cent of 400 respondents from nineteen countries acknowledged they did so, although the paper also revealed that when parents observed overt self-smelling in young children, they found it concerning and discouraged them. Paradoxically, the neurobiologist authors concluded that this behaviour has no presence in medical or psychological literature and while they suspected psychological and cultural explanations, they also argued that human self-smelling should be studied more formally by those researching social olfaction.

As happened often during my year of anosmia, I found great solace in finding slivers of information to add to my personal jigsaw but still felt the need to verify reality in my own strange world. But how could I possibly ask my husband (let alone anyone else) about this indefinable new coffee scent, let alone check its stealthy melding with the smell of poo for heaven's sake? It felt as if I was finally losing my marbles.

❋

By then, reports of coffee as a trigger of the ugly smell distortions were rife and increasing on the AbScent Facebook page and among ENT specialists seeing recovering patients. Along with onions and fried or roasted meats, it was one of the most cited suspects and was first identified, with chocolate, in one of the first studies of this kind of olfactory dysfunction, published in 2013 by the Laboratory of Neurogenetics and Behavior at New York's Rockefeller University. 'Describing odours and identifying them out of their usual context is notoriously difficult,' this report concluded, 'and this is also true for distorted odour perceptions.' One participant in the study observed 'a constant odour, not sweet not sharp, not foul, something never smelled before'; another reported, 'I started to smell coffee but not like I used to smell it. I still get these smells – also for chocolate.'[2] Oh how these words resonated.

As time passed, I became used to the off-key nature of returning smells, noting that many I'd not liked in the past were tainted with a similar, relatively pleasant, roasting-sweet-potato whiff. Cutting fresh fish from its vacuum packaging before cooking isn't always a joyous moment but this too seemed oddly benign, while dog and cat food, as it came out of the can or sachet, gave off my 'new coffee' poo smell. I laughingly nicknamed my nose distortion the 'Pollyanna parosmia' because in my world nothing smelled really, really horrible any more.

The need to sniff-test the things that I could now more easily recognise – my perfumes, essential oils, some lotions and cleansers such as shampoo or conditioner – became even more necessary. While lacking logic, in my mind the ritual felt like a reset button for my addled olfactory bulb. It would also remind me of the perfume section in large department stores where you would often see little glass bowls filled with glistening, roasted coffee beans placed beside luxurious displays of new fragrances. The idea, usually explained by a glamorous, bottle-wielding salesperson, is that if you're testing several scents at once, a sniff of the coffee beans allowed a cleansing of the 'nasal palate' or 'reset of the nose' before you moved on to the next one.

This might be a fixture in perfume retailing, but it is no more than a clever in-store marketing ploy cooked up by a couple of young Stanford graduates with degrees in bioscience and engineering. *What the Nose Knows* author Dr Avery Gilbert documented the birth of this clever selling strategy first hand as the two bright young things (who he laughingly noted 'knew beans about smell') launched an idea that would seize consumer imagination and permeate perfume marketing without an iota of scientific basis. As I read Gilbert's chapter on other, past attempts to 'reset the nose' – among them the use of vinegar rinses at nineteenth-century Japanese incense parties – I thought what a great pity it was that in reality there is no such magic bullet, given that by the European autumn, hundreds of thousands of anosmia sufferers were battling parosmia with no solution in sight.

The journal *Rhinology* published a paper that estimated that 43 per cent of patients who experienced Covid-induced smell loss were experiencing parosmia with its onset generally emerging about two and a half months after infection.[3] Judging by these statistics, I was a textbook case. Widely accepted estimates suggested that six in ten people infected with Covid-19 suffer a loss of smell or taste. This would mean that with nearly half a billion cases of infection, at the time of publication, an astounding 300 million people around the world will have experienced some kind of disturbance.

◈

Back in her University of Reading laboratory as the first lockdown eased, Dr Jane Parker and her team discovered they had more parosmia volunteers than they could manage. Where she and Chrissi Kelly had struggled to find fifteen volunteers in 2019, testing perhaps one person every couple of weeks, now they had a plethora of sufferers and a never-ending queue of guinea pigs desperate for some answers. 'People had wanted to travel to Reading from all over the world but just as supply was drying up, along came Covid,' she recalled.

Parker seized the opportunity and put her GC-O equipment back to work. Researchers had to work in full PPE kit because their volunteers, while no longer infectious, could not wear masks during the tests but the effort reaped reward pretty much straight away: the new crop's responses yielded many new and interesting observations for Parker:

> It was invaluable, this period. Before Covid we had been looking at coffee, then we got another group of participants and new triggers but we also saw some patterns in their responses; that fatigue can kick in, and that hunger can affect people's olfactory performance and the ability to recognise and identify smells was worse at those times.

Part of this is explained by 'habituation', the process by which we become less responsive to smells, usually unconsciously and most often when we are exposed to the odour continuously or repetitively. Scientists don't really know whether this occurs in a different way for every smell but Dr Parker and her team noticed that apart from habituation, tiredness definitely impacted performance.

Particularly interesting for Parker was that she could add to the shortlist of parosmia triggers collected before Covid, expanding it as more and more participants reported their experiences. They retested all the most common suspects – coffee, meat, garlic and onion – but in the second round of tests picked smells identified through a thematic analysis of posts on AbScent's Facebook parosmia page. These revealed that a particularly odd array of foods, including watermelon, cucumber, peppers and mint toothpaste, commonly triggered horrible distortions post-Covid.

Parker and Kelly worked closely with University College London ENT consultant, Simon Gane, a clinician with many years' experience working with patients suffering smell disorders. He helped explain that what makes parosmia distinctive from phantosmia is that it is triggered by an odour, lasts a relatively short time – in other words it does not linger once the source has gone – and the smell perceived is always an altered version of what you're actually smelling. 'For example, if coffee is the trigger, what you actually smell isn't what you normally recognise as coffee,' he noted, to my eternal relief. But for most people, he added, parosmia smells are almost always disgusting or unpleasant so my Pollyanna 'everything smells nice-ish' syndrome appeared to be less common.

When we first met by Zoom, Dr Parker had generously invited me to visit her lab to see the GC-O in action once lockdown and travel restrictions were eased and so, one rainy Monday morning in early spring, I got in the car and headed from London to Reading. The campus had only recently reopened to students and clutches of new returnees wandered the cafeteria and hallways, bleary-eyed as if they'd just been allowed into sunlight after a long time in the gloom of Zoom. Dr Parker led me through a labyrinth of corridors through the Food and Nutrition Science department to show me the lab's GC-O – a mysterious box with elegant innards of hair-fine wire, oven, flame and fans that could, like some kind of alchemical miracle, break smells down into their molecular components, turning the human nose into a detection device.

Over the next few hours, she showed me the vast array of odour samples prepared and sealed into small glass bottles for extraction and injection into the GC-O and ran me through the battery of tests delivered through a nose piece at timed intervals. The GC-O, after so many months idle due to Covid, insisted on glitching and so we moved on rapidly to what are universally known now as Sniffin' Sticks, devised to measure nasal chemosensory performance by Professor Gerd Kobal from Erlangen University and his then student Professor Thomas Hummel at Dresden University.

At first glance, they look like a large set of numbered fat white pens with blue caps. In fact, they are cylindrical devices with tips imbued with an array of fragrances ranging from orange, blackberry and pineapple to onion, cinnamon, anise and cigarette tobacco. These are uncapped and waved relatively briefly under your nose to test the identification of odours, discrimination between smells (via forced multiple-choice options) and odour thresholds (varying degrees of concentration from low to high until you start to perceive the smell). Dr Parker told me that ingredients are chosen to reflect cultural preferences depending on where they are being used: the German set contains the odour of sauerkraut for example, the Japanese one soy and ginger.

It took more than an hour to work through three sets of twenty-five sticks using what is described as the staircase method, which means that two of the three sticks are blank or are stronger/easier to detect until you recognise the smell but then, once you get it right, you are offered sticks at smell levels that make it more difficult again. It turned out to be a remarkably tiring exercise and I felt nervous and anxious throughout, worried about what my scores might show and just how badly my fifth sense might have eroded.

Thankfully, as her first guinea pig out of lockdown, my discrimination/identification scores turned out to be decent – great news for my recovery from anosmia – although the threshold tests were not great. Intrigued by my response to coffee/poo, Dr Parker pledged to bring me back to the lab once the GC-O was returned to full health. A quick visit to show me the department's 'fume hood' – an air-locked cupboard where the stinkiest samples are diluted to minuscule proportions – made me wonder at the time about the wisdom of this future commitment.

Ultimately, a return would not be necessary because within months, Dr Parker's study and comparison between those suffering distortions and the control group with a normal sense of smell would confirm, for the first time, that not only is there a molecular basis for parosmia but that it is not linked to the ability to smell and can occur even in those suffering anosmia.[4] In fact, the team identified 15 different molecular triggers in coffee and whittled the trigger culprits down to two major groups of molecules, one containing sulphur and one containing nitrogen atoms. Both these groups share a very low odour threshold in humans and are found in a vast array of different foods.

Interestingly, the most frequently reported trigger, known rather forgettably as 2-furanmethanethiol, is the one that imparts the roasted, coffee-like flavour. It has a particularly low odour threshold when diluted in water, making it one of the most detectable. While normal subjects described it as 'roasty', a little like popcorn, or even smoky, to those with impaired smell like me, it wasn't perceptible in the same way and could be described only as 'new coffee' or for many others, simply disgusting, dirty or repulsive.

The mysterious nature of the fifth sense was underlined in many other ways by the results of Parker's studies. For example, one person suffered parosmia that was not preceded by anosmia, much like Sir David Hare's experience. This participant identified around forty-five different aromas but only two turned out to be triggers for distortions. Another subject altogether found their parosmia improved dramatically but without any increase in smell function, while another, rather happier case who had suffered parosmia for several years, reported dramatic improvements and scored well on the Sniffin' Sticks tests.

For me, however, it was the group's findings on faecal odours that were the most intriguing. It seems some parosmic participants often commented to the researchers that the smell of poo never seemed as unpleasant as they remembered it or that it smelled like other foods, certainly more pleasant and often slightly 'biscuity'. This presented Parker's team with the odd corollary that foods smell of faeces and yet faeces smell of food – exactly what I'd encountered. As Professor Barry Smith described it, quoting Macbeth, 'fair is foul and foul is fair'.

To test this, during the study, two parosmic members of the research team and one person from the normal control group volunteered for the hideous job of sniffing a mix of 50 per cent faecal slurry via the GC-O. While the person with normal smell gagged and perceived the strongest imaginable intensity of poo smell (thanks to the culprit molecules, indole, skatole and p-cresol), the parosmics simply didn't register the foul smell, reporting only the triggers already mentioned in coffee.

This, according to Parker's study, provides a neat explanation for the odd reversal of foul to fair smell among those with parosmia: if you perceive only some molecules and not others then poo smells different. In the absence of signals from the usual stinky compounds found in poo, participants like me detected some of the other potent volatiles, ones that in turn were normally masked by the smelliest ones for those with a normal sense of smell. In the end, the way parosmics perceive poo depends on their sensitivity to the other array of odour molecules present.

As is so often the case in science, answering one question leads to the need to ask another. This study has now placed a great big question mark on earlier theories that parosmia is the result of neuronal mis-wiring during regeneration after injury such as a virus or brain trauma. While the team showed that the olfactory distortions have a molecular basis, it has not been able to identify the specific olfactory receptors responsible despite conducting a deep dive into publicly available databases. The fact that some participants reported distortion with only some of the molecule groups suggests that there may be up to four separate olfactory receptors involved – perhaps even more when other food and household items such as cleaning sprays that elicit distortions were added to the mix.

'The more you look', observed Parker, 'the more difficult and complex and interesting it becomes.'

14

A Bunch of Little Sadnesses

There was little understanding of smell loss, let alone parosmia back in 2009 when Katie Boateng, creator and host of The Smell Podcast, realised she had lost her fifth sense. Katie was a college student near her home town in southern Idaho when one of her flatmates began to clean the table around her while she ate her breakfast cereal. Irritated by the idea of a powerful chemical being sprayed while she was eating, she asked her flatmate to stop but in that moment noticed that despite its proximity she couldn't smell the bleach at all.

Puzzled, she immediately walked around their shared apartment, sniffing anything she could find but perceiving nothing. Katie had been laid low by a respiratory virus a few weeks earlier, but hadn't thought too much about it until then. She decided to make an appointment with the family doctor when she returned home for the summer holidays. He later confirmed that the virus was most probably the culprit for her smell loss and prescribed a course of nasal steroids in the meantime while also warning that she would need patience while her olfactory system recovered. Several months passed with no improvement, prompting Katie to ask for a referral to an ENT specialist who ordered a CT scan to rule out tumours and conducted a full examination of her nasal cavity in case of chronic disease such as polyps or rhinusitis:

> The tests all came back clear and I was then referred to a neurologist for brain-related issues. When those tests showed nothing too, that was that . . . I can see now, looking back, that this was the most difficult time for me. It was the end of the road, there didn't seem to be anything else that they could offer and I'd never imagined that I might not get better.
>
> There were no support services available and I don't even remember the word anosmia being used to explain what had happened . . . perhaps the ENT mentioned it once?

Katie found herself alone with a new sensory reality she did not understand and had certainly not expected. She believes that for seven or eight years she went into a kind of denial, simply ignoring her condition, sealing the problem 'into a box' that she steadfastly refused to open.

> I finished my degree, in Spanish-language teaching, taught high school and later got married. I think it was just too painful for me to think about what I had lost for a long time but that's really how I got to start the podcast. Years later, when we moved to New Jersey for my husband's job, I was looking for work and so I had more time on my hands. I love listening to podcasts, they are one of my favourite things to do along with reading and I decided I wanted to

create something for people that might have been useful to me back in 2009.

Katie says that when she launched the podcast in August 2018, she didn't really know what she was doing, reaching out to people online to ask if they would share their experience with her and learning as she went along. Now she is a founding member of and works part-time for STANA, the newly formed Smell and Taste Association of North America. When I discovered the podcast, Katie was onto her eightieth episode, interviewing a host of interesting and diverse people who have lived with an array of olfactory disruptions. I immersed myself in a binge-fest of her interviews and every day, walking the dog, I'd put on my headphones and listen to experiences in the unpredict-able world of olfactory distortion, becoming increasingly more familiar with the condition as the conversations with her guests described their lives.

'In life, I have always asked myself the question, "Why not me?"' Katie told me as we chatted across time zones. 'So I thought, why don't I make a podcast?' Katie's work over the last few years has created a unique audio library of the experi-ences of anosmic and parosmic people – some who were born without a sense of smell; others who had lost it through illness or trauma – explaining how they perceive the world and the ways they navigate day-to-day life without the fifth sense. Along with wide-ranging interviews with neuroscientists and chemosensory researchers, psychologists, philosophers, writers and chefs, it is an excellent digital resource for anyone interested in the olfactory world but invaluable for anosmics.

Katie, like Chrissi Kelly, had an instinctive response as Covid took off and was quick to note anecdotal evidence of a potential link between anosmia and the new virus. On 24 March 2020 she devoted her weekly programme to reading aloud an article written for *Forbes* magazine by an infectious diseases specialist, Dr Judy Stone, that flagged the possibility that Covid might well be responsible for olfactory loss.

In her interviews, Katie often asks her guests what they miss most about the sense of smell. While we chatted, it seemed right to ask her the same question. What she said and the sadness of her tone surprised me:

> A huge part of my universe is missing and much of that, I think, is linked to memory. There is a lot of research now about the links between smell and memory and I've become convinced that mine has got a lot worse since I had anosmia. I can't remember things in the same way . . . I can't walk into a Bath and Bodyworks shop and smell the perfume that used to transport me back to junior high . . . it was a cucumber and melon spray that all my friends and I lathered on when we were all together. I can't have that feeling that transports you to those moments.

Another example she pointed out is one I could also relate to viscerally: the smell of clean laundry, fresh out of the dryer or brought inside from the line after being outside in the sunshine.

> This happened to me a couple of months ago and when I remembered that it's not an experience I can have any

more, I cried. Of course, I am fine, I have adapted, I get on with life. But what I would like people to know is that with anosmia, there are a lot of little sadnesses. I am happy with my life but sometimes it is hard to be reminded of the loss.

Katie is quick to add that she does not expect or imagine that her experience is universal for all anosmics, knowing through listening to others that some miss certain things very much while others don't.

I don't want to be an authority on how you should feel something and if you don't feel you're missing out that is valid too. My goal with sharing stories is that we all know we are not alone, that others are going through something similar and to compare and share these stories is what I find extremely comforting.

Katie is now in a second decade without her fifth sense and says that while she is resilient, has adapted and learned to cope well, every now and then she also gets caught off guard emotionally: 'Bam! It happens out of nowhere. I'd like people to understand just how sad and upsetting these little moments can be.'

If someone came along with a magic wand and offered to restore her olfactory system, would she go ahead? Katie's answer surprised me again: I'd want it if it came back, yes – but I would want it to work perfectly. I have interviewed so many people who have had parosmia and it can be horrific.

I would not want to go through that and I would not want it back if it meant that. Of course, it would be beautiful if it came back, overwhelming, and it would take me time to get used to it again. Perhaps it might even be scary as I tried to understand what was happening my brain. Also I met my husband after I got anosmia: I don't know how he smells and what if I didn't like it?

She laughed. 'I guess I'd just have to get used to it.'

＊

Across the Atlantic in London, Louise Woollam is also no stranger to anosmia. Rather than creating a podcast about her experience, she felt driven to write about it. It was the spring of 2014 when she caught a heavy cold and, after a fortnight of congestion, realised her condition was rather more serious than merely stuffed-up sinuses. Louise had completely lost her sense of smell.

Apart from confusion with a condition that nobody seemed able to explain or remedy, Louise had another reason to be distressed by the turn of events. Away from her job as an accountant with a charity, she had established a successful side career as a culture writer, cranking out witty and acerbic observations several times a week from her front room. Louise had launched her beauty blog, Get Lippie in 2009 and it had morphed naturally into a series of columns focused on the art of perfumery and fragrances. It had quickly gained an audience and soon she was being nominated for writing awards, most notably by the perfume industry body the Fragrance Foundation.

Then came anosmia.

It would take several months before Louise was able to secure an appointment with an ENT specialist. She was prescribed a course of steroids and told to be patient and return for a check-up in six months. But, by then, what started as a smell vacuum had deteriorated into a roller-coaster of distortions and phantom smells, turning what already felt like a bad dream into an unbearable reality. Chocolate biscuits tasted like burned leaves and mould; she had a constant smell of smoke in her nostrils and paradoxically found herself desperate for flavour, even smothering orange and chocolate Jaffa cakes with hot sauce in a desperate attempt to get a hit of something tasty.

Leaving the house each morning to travel into central London for work became almost impossible: walking past a Starbucks next to her office, she felt as if she was hitting a wall of sewage, so awful was the distorted smell of coffee. The waft of cigarette smoke in the street overpowered her senses and made her gag, while the clash of deodorants, colognes and perfumes exuded by workmates in the office made her head spin. Eventually, she stopped commuting and retreated to her home, which was the only place she felt she could control her olfactory environment.

Worry slowly turned to despair and bouts of depression, heightened when one specialist made an off-hand comment about a famous rock star who had become anosmic and ended his own life. 'It was the last thing I needed to hear,' she recalled with some bitterness. Louise was lucky and a breakthrough came unexpectedly around six months after falling ill when she decided, despite her condition, to attend a perfume writers' tour of the Osmothèque in Versailles, the world's largest scent archive. She and fellow perfume writers on the tour were led through the museum to sniff dozens of the most iconic fragrances created from the end of the nineteenth century.

They began with the aromatic citrus of *Eau de Lubin*, working through the lavender and bergamot of *Fougère Royale*, the vanilla spice of *L'Heure Bleue* and the musky rose of Jean Patou's *Joy*. Louise either smelled nothing or a distortion until the moment when she passed her nose over *Vera Violetta*, created in 1894 by the perfumer Roger & Gallet:

> I realised that what I could smell wasn't a booze-soaked pig who'd been rolling in icing sugar, like some of the previous fragrances, but actual, real and undistorted violets. This was the first thing I'd smelled at all, never mind *correctly*, in over six months. That first, ever-so-faint and rather prickly smell of violet was probably the most beautiful thing I've ever had near my nose. I hadn't realised just how dark, and unfulfilled, a life either without smell entirely, or a life with only bad things to smell had been until then.

Buoyed by the response and surprised that she was smelling elements of citrus by the end of the tour, Louise decided to experiment by using her own collection of hundreds of bottles of perfume stashed around her house to try to retrain her sense of smell, wearing a different fragrance each day and then writing a short note and posting it on Instagram under #LipsNspritz.

It was instinct rather than advice that drove her idea and yet it turned out to be the right thing to do. Many of the perfumes held no smell and others were distorted but, as she persisted, the experiment began to work; the smells, however disgusting at first, began to evolve as her brain and nose worked together to relearn the fragrances. Louise would post more than 400 times over the next two years:

> Smell training is like learning a new language. A lot of people get this mixed up with aromatherapy because they use essential oils but in my mind, smell training is nothing to do with the way things actually smell; rather it's about taking the time to retrain your brain to think about smell and hopefully regenerate your library of smells.
>
> You don't understand the language or the grammar until you immerse yourself into it. Take lemons as an example; think about the associations of the smells, like an amazing holiday or a lemon-flavoured cocktail rather than the smell itself. You can't just break down the smell to its constituent parts and expect to relearn it.

Once she had started, Louise realised very quickly that the more often she encountered something – even something that was disgusting initially – the more easily she was able to distinguish 'that particular *something*' and that the smell improved incrementally each time.

> Even with things like coffee, and chocolate, and bacon, which were my worst triggers for a long time. Tempting though it is for a parosmic to retreat into a 'safe' world of beige and white food that doesn't cause reactions, and to avoid fragrances and try to live as smell-lessly as possible, I think that can just exacerbate the issue. It's counter-intuitive, I know, that the answer to things smelling disgusting might

159

actually be to smell *more* disgusting things, and more often, but I think it's definitely helped me.

Even so, there were still smells that remained out of reach and Louise wasn't afraid to experiment: 'People go on about what smell they would most miss – coffee or new-born baby's head. Well, I missed the smell of my own farts,' she laughed.

I must admit that I did not share this particular nostalgia with her but what Louise did next intrigued me. She decided to collect a range of perfumes known for their indolic and skatolic components to see if she could train herself to smell poo again:

I picked ten fragrances from the 'somebody farted in the next room' through to 'the sewerage farm next to the manure pile' range. Not only could I smell poo better at the end of it but the feature I wrote about it was nominated for another award.

Louise has regained about 80 per cent of smell in her right nostril but the left nostril remains a blank. Her husband had been very supportive during her ordeal, even learning to cook because she couldn't stand being in the kitchen: 'He smelled like Bisto gravy powder but he's gone back to smelling like Parma ham now,' she quipped before becoming more serious:

You don't realise how much you rely on your sense of smell until you lose it. Showering isn't the same, brushing your teeth isn't the same, meeting other people isn't the same. I think we are taught to ignore our sense of smell to an extent. We don't think about it and we don't have language for it, so people simply don't realise that 100 per cent of the time they are smelling stuff.

Because of the way the brain works, looking for novel smells and filtering out normal smells, you just don't realise that you are smelling all of the time. But the second something changes in your vicinity you notice it, like someone burning toast in another room, because that's the way the brain processes it. Your nose is in your line of vision all the time and yet the brain filters it out so you don't see it.

She has given lectures at the Royal Society of Medicine, spoken at a European Rhinologists' conference and helped fundraise for the UK anosmia charity Fifth Sense by creating and selling a scent called *Paradox* combining lemon petitgrain, irises and violets in a collaboration with perfumer Sarah McCartney of 4160 Tuesdays.

Despite the new attention on anosmia and its variants, Louise remains concerned that the NHS has no recognised pathways for people who lose their sense of smell: 'An artist with vision problems can get a referral to a specialist but there isn't anything like that for a person without smell or taste. There should be.'

15

My Designated Nose

Robert here. I am taking over narration, if only briefly.

Paola has long told me that she doesn't think I have a great sense of smell. Looking back, I think it could be the result of childhood surgery back in the 1960s when I had my tonsils and adenoids removed. (Adenoids are glands that form part of the body's immune system, helping to protect against viruses and bacteria. In the past, they were often removed when they became swollen or enlarged in young children hindering breathing and speech.) Whatever the reason, in our house Paola has been the setter of scent standards, choosing the flowers, reminding me to open windows when cooking, hunting out socks stuffed inside running shoes that needed washing and detecting that the dog might need his butt fur tended to. Annoyingly, even before I'd walked through the front door she could sniff out the occasional cigarette I'd sneaked in the days I struggled to give up the appalling habit. But all that changed on 27 March 2020, when her sudden anosmia forced a role reversal, and the nasal dullard of the family – *moi* – suddenly became the designated nose. I was the airport drug hound, unleashed to provide olfactory confirmation as she struggled to come to terms with a world that had become instantly oblique. Paola's joy in cooking and the subtle flavours of her Neapolitan heritage had been reduced to sight and guesswork rather than refinement of taste from the bubbling saucepan. Dinner-table conversations began with doubts and questions: was there enough salt, could I taste the basil?

I have to admit here that I enjoyed the freedom it gave me to cook meat and fish without comment from the floors above that I had stunk out the kitchen. Having said that, I am reminded of the two fillet steaks I found and bought in the first week of lockdown as supermarkets emptied in the ensuing panic-buying. When I suggested them for dinner, Paola gagged at the very thought of meat, its texture impossible to manage without flavour. The steaks remained frozen until fifteen months later when I found them during a clean-out, like some ancient Arctic discovery. The other immediate challenge was personal hygiene, as Paola was reluctantly forced to trust her husband's assurances that she didn't smell of body odour – not that she ever did.

Dog walks, already governed by our scent-driven Cairn terrier's insistence on pausing to smell every trace of other dogs, became even longer as Paola stopped frequently to stick her head in a bush, hoping to get a hint of spring flowers. My reluctant confirmation of the scent of jasmine that she couldn't detect just cemented her frustration. It was hard to watch. It's not that I had no understanding of her situation. We'd had Covid at the same time and the morning after her smell loss, I went downstairs to make bacon and egg sandwiches for brunch – a favourite culinary offering I take pride in on the weekend. Paola chewed her 'sarnie' reluctantly, grateful for the varying textures and combination but, missing the taste of bacon and bread and noticing mainly the salt, it was a muted joy. When I returned to the kitchen to enjoy my creation, it was horrific. The bread was like chewing on cardboard – tasteless and flat. I still recall it more than a year later. I was lucky, the smell loss partial and lasting a few days at most, but enough to get a hint of Paola's new, scentless world. Things changed again a few months later when her sense of smell began to return. She shrieked with delight one morning when she stopped at the jasmine bush along the dog walk, inhaled deeply and detected a hint of its spicy sweetness. This time I was happy to make the confirmation.

When she developed a smell lock and was plagued by the waft of charcoal, it seemed to me that her olfactory world had become pixilated; like a badly tuned TV she required constant checks about whether smells were real or imagined.

In the midst of lockdown we had developed some easy, bowl dinners that could be eaten in front of the television and away from the nightly temptation of a glass of wine. My bastardised kedgeree was one of our favourites, a quick mix of smoked mackerel, onions, peas, rice and cubes of roasted sweet potato. Chilli mackerel was our favourite, as it seemed to blast through the anosmia to some degree although there was one drawback – for Paola, the smell of roasting sweet potato had also become disturbingly similar to what we politely call bathroom smells.

At the time of writing, the nasal pixilation remains a challenge with Paola unable to trust the sense of smell that is returning in bits and pieces. I am reminded of this every morning when we have our first espresso to start the day. 'It's the ritual and sweetness,' she tells me when I ask. 'Coffee has a new smell but I can't tell you what it is. It smells like poo but then poo doesn't smell like poo any more either.'

*

I had an easy time of it compared to the experience of Matt Wallace, the partner of smell-blighted perfume writer Louise Woollam. Although she tends to make light of her situation, or at least soften the experience with humour, it is clear from Matt's recollection that the onset of anosmia had a devastating impact emotionally as well as physically. As a result, his role was not only important from a practical perspective, negotiating the world of no smells and then phantom ones, but also as a psychological support. The lack of answers about her condition left his wife increasingly worried, angry and tearful. With the onset of parosmia and phantosmia, he found himself parrying a barrage of questions he simply could not answer, unable to appreciate fully the awful smells, real and imagined, that Louise had to deal with from day to day:

> Reactions to everyday things became more extreme – washing her hair made her sick, as did the smell of cigarettes, coffee, other things. Conversations revolved around situations that had happened at work, on the street, about how she was having to have uncomfortable and often awkward conversations with uncomprehending people.
>
> Days when there had been an event of some perfume kind varied massively. If she had had to have a conversation with someone, it was humiliating. Obviously we talked, we

worked it through, and we tried to work out if there was a
way to avoid it the next day. It was much crisis management
and trying to get by day by day.

Cooking, a recurring issue with anosmics and their partners, presented its own set of problems. The challenge for Matt was to
create meals with texture:

> It was a bonus if Louise could taste any hint of flavour.
> Hot sauces became a staple, regardless of what was
> being cooked – more important on the table than salt and
> pepper.

Things changed again – and dramatically – when parosmia
kicked in:

> Grilling anything – meat or vegetables – became almost
> impossible because the slightest hint of carbonised mater-
> ial overwhelmed Louise with burnt flavours and sensations.
> Unless it could be smothered or disguised, it had to be
> something safe. Even now, we tend to avoid mixing sauces
> through a meal, such as pasta sauces, in case there's an
> adverse reaction or the taste becomes overwhelming.

The impact was more than just dealing with food. Her love of
perfume became a trigger for her situation:

> There was the frustration of losing the sense that had
> allowed her passion to write about perfume. She feared

losing everything associated with it – the friends, the events, the whole passion being snuffed out – so it became difficult and painful to even discuss anything to do with perfume.

It remains a challenge, he says, even though Louise has recovered her sense of smell to some extent:

> She can lead a mostly 'normal' life, and extreme parosmic events are very rare. Bad days are few and far between, and we are back to eating almost everything we feel like, without having to worry about things. However, she is nowhere near recovered enough in order to feel comfortable venturing back into the world of perfume events and writing without it generally being related in some way to her condition. A couple of perfumers have been incredibly helpful in terms of doing things like smell training and working with Louise to see what she can smell and what smells 'nice', but it feels like her confidence to re-engage with that side of blogging and writing is gone.

When Katie Price met Stephen Boateng in 2009 she too was struggling to come to terms with her anosmia but was worried and reluctant about discussing it in detail with her new boyfriend: 'Katie told me at the time that she didn't have a sense of smell and was going back to her home town to be diagnosed by the family doctor,' Stephen told me. 'But she didn't like talking too much about it because she was trying to figure out what it meant to her,' he recalled.

Taking his anosmic girlfriend out for a romantic dinner would be one of the first challenges, a time when impressions count most in a fledgling relationship. Stephen says he tried to focus on conversation and companionship to compensate: 'The goal for me was to focus on us being together and enjoying each other's company rather than the meal itself.' As time passed however, and they became more comfortable with each other – and the situation – they were able to venture into new territory. 'At the table and when the smell of a specific food came up, we would use that as an opportunity for Katie to share any frustrations she might be feeling about it.'

There would also be funny moments, like the time during a family event that Katie joked that at least she couldn't tell if Stephen smelled badly: 'Her sisters and her mom insisted that I actually smelled good. Katie laughed and said something like, "I'm happy you all are able to smell him for me."'

On a practical level, Stephen has found himself being vigilant in reminding her about doing smell training and is also her sentinel to ensure food like fruit and vegetables or leftovers from dinner in refrigerator are still okay to eat. 'Sometimes it can be difficult to know if food is okay to eat just by looking at it so if it's been a while she will ask me to smell it to make sure.' Katie's anosmia, he says, means she has lost much of the joy of cooking but for him that is easy to manage: 'I really do enjoy cooking so I am able to do that for both of us. I don't view her anosmia as an issue and I enjoy coming up with new recipes for us to enjoy together.'

But of all the help, Stephen says his wife's podcast has been the most positive influence on her struggles with the disability:

It's always good to know that there are other people out in the world who can relate to your own experiences. The podcast guests are like an extended family to her. Everyone deals and copes with their anosmia differently. What's important to me is to find out what works for Katie as she goes about her day while living with anosmia. Anosmia is only a small part of her story but it doesn't define her. The fact that she can cope with it by creating the podcast is amazing.

PART 3

16

The Devil Inside

It was an innocent summer evening of bicycles, beer and pizza that would end in the tragic alteration of a young man's life. In the summer of 1992 Michael Hutchence, the sensual lead singer of Australian band INXS, was riding his bike home from a night out in Copenhagen with his girlfriend, supermodel Helena Christensen, when they stopped to buy a pizza. Michael carried the box and wobbled as he pedalled unsteadily down the middle of a narrow cobbled side street towards Christensen's apartment in the historic centre of the city. He stopped halfway down the street, opened the box and began eating a slice, still perched on the bike, just as a taxi entered the same street and drove up behind the pair. Annoyed that he couldn't get around the cyclists, the driver beeped his horn and yelled. When Hutchence didn't move, the man got out of his car and confronted him. Neither backed down and during an altercation, the driver, whom Christensen later described as crazy, lashed out and punched Hutchence, who reeled back and fell, striking his head on the pavement. It was the moment that his family and friends believe ultimately led to his suicide five years later.

That night in Copenhagen Hutchence lay unconscious on the road, blood running from his mouth, nose and ears. 'I thought he was dead,' Christensen recalled in the 2019 documentary *Mystify*. An ambulance was called and took him to hospital where the singer was checked and released in a matter of hours, even though he was acting erratically. 'They thought he was drunk and wanted to go. It was a mistake,' she said. A week later Hutchence was still hiding in Christensen's apartment where he was ill and vomiting blood. 'I would bring him food but he would push it away, sometimes almost violently.'

It would be another month before he was persuaded to see doctors in Paris who discovered that he had two large contusions and permanent damage to his frontal lobes. The olfactory neurones had been severed, which meant he had lost his sense of smell. But the report would remain confidential and Christensen was sworn to secrecy by Hutchence even as his moods changed and his enjoyment of life disappeared. Before the accident, Christensen said he was intoxicatingly sweet, funny and emotional but he had now become erratic, angry, often confused and increasingly dejected as a succession of experts told him it would be impossible to reconnect the nerve: 'He broke down and told me, "I'll never be able to smell my baby when I have a child." Things just got really heavy.'

Friends, family and fellow band members watched with increasing concern the changes in his behaviour, which manifested in frequent angry explosions followed by bouts of sadness, tears and incoherence.

'When Michael hit his head, he came back a different person,' the band's bass guitarist Garry Beers told Australian television in 2014. 'It wasn't the Michael we knew and that's what was so surprising. He couldn't smell and he couldn't taste, he was drinking wine by the bottle cos it was just like nothing to him. He was quite clearly suffering from serious brain damage.'

Lead guitarist Tim Farriss also saw the changes: 'You never knew what you were going to get from day to day. One day you would get [the old] Michael and the next this aggressive, violent monster. It was like dealing with bipolar. He was very erratic in his behaviour but also what we were trying to do musically.'

His personal manager Martha Troup could see more deeply, beyond his day-to-day struggles with food and drink:

> He confessed to me that it changed everything. What was just a sweet insecurity became a deep insecurity. He kind of lost his way and forgot who he was. To lose the sense that really gives you that primal sense of hedonism was really devastating to someone who was already engineered that way . . . It was like floating in outer space; you can still see and hear things but there is this absence and emptiness. And it gets worse over time, not better.

Hutchence once attempted to describe the frustration: 'I spent about a year doing what I call sensitising. It's like taking your knuckles and rubbing them raw to feel things. Not just having knowledge, but feeling . . . really feeling.' An indication of Hutchence's sensory despair was poignantly illustrated by his passion and fascination for the 1985 novel *Perfume* by the German writer Patrick Süskind, possibly the most vivid exploration of the fifth sense and its connection with the most visceral emotions told through the fictional story of the eighteenth-century perfumer turned murderer Jean-Baptiste Grenouille.[1] Long before his accident, Hutchence had delighted in giving a copy of the book to his then lover, fellow Australian singer Kylie Minogue. The couple spent the early hours of one morning exploring the streets of Paris to find places mentioned in the novel. Minogue recorded her lover's delight as he retold her the plot. The intimate recording, featured in the *Mystify* documentary, shows a young man clearly intimately connected with his fifth sense, elated by what it brought to his creativity, imagination, connection with other:

> Grenouille smells everything so acutely . . . but he doesn't have a smell of his own, so he makes his own smell but it's not good enough. Then one day, he smells this smell, so he follows the scent from the Right Bank to the Left Bank in Paris and he comes to a young virgin who smells like peaches. He has never seen beauty like it, never known a woman. He makes twenty perfumes from twenty virgins until he is the most notorious murderer in the world. He escapes to the mountains where they grow all the flowers to make all the perfume in the world . . . He is the greatest perfumer in all of the world but eventually he goes back to say sorry. But they catch him and all of Paris goes insane. They are going to behead him but he has one last wish: 'Give me my bag' and he puts all the perfumes into one. The whole city goes into an orgy and they tear him apart.

In July 1996 Hutchence had a daughter with the television presenter Paula Yates. He adored the child. In November 1997 he travelled to Australia to embark on a twentieth-anniversary tour with INXS, buoyed by the expectation that Yates and the children would soon be joining him.

On the night of 21 November, Yates phoned to say that her trip had been cancelled. Sir Bob Geldof, Yates's husband and the father of her elder daughters, had taken legal action to stop her from taking the children out of the country. Alone in a room at the Ritz-Carlton Hotel in Double Bay, Sydney, Hutchence phoned Geldof to protest. The next morning, Hutchence was found dead, hanged by his snakeskin belt buckled to the door knob.

Filmmaker Richard Lowenstein, who made the *Mystify* documentary and was a close friend of Hutchence, was able to gain access to the coroner's report, which revealed the extent of the damage to the singer's brain and olfactory system. The coroner, Derrick Hand, concluded that a combination of depression, alcohol, stress and sleeplessness had created a toxic cocktail and led to Hutchence's decision to end his own life.

※

Michael Hutchence's growing and inescapable feelings of sadness, his difficulty sleeping and his loss of appetite are all key symptoms in the clinical diagnosis of depression. Today we know that many sufferers of anosmia have similar experiences. Laboratory studies with rats that have had their olfactory bulbs surgically removed to ensure they cannot smell reveal that the animals develop behavioural as well as physiological changes similar to those seen in human patients with significant depressive illness.[2]

Their feeding behaviours change, their learning abilities become less effective, and their motivation to move around in the cage reduces. Anosmic rats' interest in social interaction and play slumps and they also show greater stress responses when introduced to novel environments, affecting short-term memory and sleep cycles. When treated with common antidepressant medication such as Serotonin Reuptake Inhibitors, symptoms were alleviated. While the link between smell loss and depression in humans is correlational, there have been a multitude of studies over the past decade to test and verify the connection in clinical settings.

Kim Price lives with her husband on the edge of the New Forest. A passionate nature lover, she lost her sense of smell and taste ten years ago after hitting her head when she fell from a ladder. Kim spent several days in intensive care and in a chemically induced coma. It took a long time to recover and while she realised that she had lost her sense of smell early on, the severity of her injury led her into a state of denial about her loss for more than three years: 'The journey for those who get anosmia from traumatic injury is very different to others, particularly when we talk about loss caused by Covid-19,' she told me. 'There are so many other things going on, between recovery and rehabilitation, that smell ends up a long way down on the priority list.'

Kim told a nurse while she was still in hospital that she couldn't smell and has never forgotten the knowing nod of acknowledgment – not reassurance – that she received in return: 'From that, I picked up that there wasn't necessarily going to be an answer or a cure for me.' Kim went through a long, roller-coaster of grief. 'It's a very personal loss and it's very hard to explain what it is like. Sometimes, for example, I wish they would rewrite the dictionary and all entries on smell and taste,' she told me. 'People say to me, "Well you can still taste at least." No, I cannot. I cannot perceive flavours.'

It took Kim about three and a half years to recover fully physically. Her battle to come to terms with her anosmia took even longer and, in some ways, is still ongoing:

Because I was so grateful to survive the injury and what was a near-death experience, I just put it into a box and didn't think about it because I almost felt it was insignificant. My family, friends, so many people would say, 'Well, at least you can see and hear.' I'd go, 'Yeah', and say to myself, 'Get a grip', and then enter a circle of guilt about it. I can see now that I was starting to struggle psychologically.

In the end, Kim realised that she was falling into a dark place and contacted her GP who fortunately sent her back to a specialist liaison nurse at the hospital where she had originally been treated. Despite feeling guilty and even a little ashamed about surviving a life-threatening injury and 'returning with a complaint', Kim took the GP's advice:

I had been very aware of smell and life was all about the fragrance of flowers and nature, about the smell of clean laundry, about food, about the seasons. So when I sat down and she asked me how I'd been I just broke down about not being able to smell or taste. Until then, I had no idea how big this was for me, no idea. The very key thing she told me

was to treat it as a bereavement. To hear that said was a hal-
lelujah moment: number one that somebody was taking this
seriously and number two acknowledging that it is a loss. It
is a huge loss. Part of you wants to put it in a box, forget the
terrible sense of what is missing and just not be reminded.

The relief Kim felt at having her grief recognised and legitimised
is palpable more than a decade later. I understood too her sense
of guilt about complaining about the loss of smell, having felt
exactly the same shame talking about it when so many people
were suffering and dying as Covid swept the world.

I wondered if she, like Michael Hutchence, had succumbed
to moments of anger in the wake of her injury and smell loss
but she says this is not in her natural disposition. For her it is a
deep sadness that she still needs to keep at bay, committing to
cardiovascular exercise every other day for physical and mental
health and taking time and extra care preparing food for balanced
nutrition.

'I describe my anosmia as an invisible, heart-breaking torture,
almost impossible to share or articulate. The closest I can get to it
is: "What does silence sound like? What does nothing look like?"'
Kim says she instinctively feels that Hutchence's decision to keep
his anosmia secret from his friends and loved ones would have
compounded his loss. Physical and mental exhaustion, anger and
confusion are all recognised aspects of recovering from brain
injury and ongoing sensory loss, and the absence of support adds
to psychological turmoil. Kim makes the point that olfactory
dysfunction is a serious condition for those affected by it and
it deserves much more attention from doctors and health care

professionals who treat affected patients, as well as from scientists who research treatment options.

She is adamant that anosmia triggers anhedonia, the inability to experience pleasure and often described as the 'why does nothing feel good any more' syndrome. Kim says when the beautiful nuances of smell and flavour go, so do many other joys:

> There is a lack of anticipation, arousal, and stimulation, a lack of satiation. I can't help but feel robbed of a world I once knew, it's an incredibly personal loss. It's so important to try and fill in the gaps. I confess it's not always easy. It's important to share your feelings with a trusted friend, family member, doctor or health care professional.

Taking pleasure from food colours and textures from all the important food groups is hugely important to Kim and she experiments with different ways to enjoy the rituals of preparing and sharing dishes with friends and family. She laughs a little sadly when she tells me how much she misses the simplest pleasures such as baked beans on toast but adds quickly that she has learned to be kind to herself, turning to nature and the outdoors to fill some of the gaps left by smell:

> It's important to look after yourself. To give people hope that as time goes on the loss becomes more normal – you don't feel the absence as much every single time you are reminded of it. Not being able to smell my husband is so desperately sad, the smell of a new country when you walk out of the airport, the smell of shampoos and lotions in

the shower . . . thank goodness the brain does accept with time and then you go for other angles, you try to feel the texture of the shampoo, to have crisp linen in the bedroom, you compensate.

There was a time in the early years, she adds, when she used to dream that someone famous who had experienced anosmia might seek the public spotlight to talk about it, give it a platform:

Of course I didn't mean this in a nasty way: I wouldn't wish it on anyone but I racked my brains for many years to find a way to get it out there, to get people to understand what it means when you lose your sense of smell. And of course now, Covid has done that.

I hope it will also bring more attention and understanding.

17

The Grandfather
of Olfaction

There is probably no one who knows more about the sense of smell than Professor Thomas Hummel and his wife, Dr Cornelia Hummel. They have been studying the human olfactory system – and anosmia – for forty years and, between them, published more than 500 scientific papers. Cornelia was among the first to record electro-physiological evidence of the perception of odours in humans in the late 1980s. In 1998, Thomas founded and still heads the world-renowned Smell and Taste Clinic at the Carl Gustav Carus University in Dresden, Germany. Among his own list of extraordinary achievements was a collaboration, with his supervisor, pharmacology professor Gerd Kobal, that led to the invention of the so-called Sniffin' Sticks, the system of odour-coded pens now used globally by clinicians to test nasal chemosensory performance, although Hummel chose deliberately not to take any financial interest in their manufacture and sale.

Thomas Hummel has trained a generation of olfactory researchers and clinicians. Every year a new crop comes from every corner of the globe to spend time in the clinic's laboratories or to work with the patients who seek help for smell and gustatory problems. Often described as the grandfather of olfaction studies, in real life Thomas could be the research scientist from Central Casting, reading glasses hung precariously in his top pocket and a white moustache even more luxuriant than Albert Einstein's. Thomas and his collaborators have added innumerable, important layers of understanding about the physiology of smell and taste function, not just documenting perception but linking olfaction with mood and emotion, revealing that brain structures themselves can change when smell is lost or disrupted, and also testing and collecting evidence about techniques that can help regain function.

Cornelia Hummel's pioneering work with electroencephalography (EEG) was published in 1988[1] and she later moved on to magnetic source imaging (MSI) and magnetoencephalography (MEG), recording the magnetic field emitted by neurones. Cornelia and her team documented the brain's responses to non-invasive stimuli (known in laboratory speak as 'event-related potentials') and were able to map for the first time the specific neo-cortical areas within the brain's limbic system that light up and respond to smell – in their test case the odours of hydrogen sulphide and vanillin.

In humans, we know that the limbic system, driver of the behavioural responses needed for survival, emerged from the olfactory bulb, the most primitive of the brain structures. This formed the neural hard-wiring that fuels our fight and flight responses, hunger (and protective responses to toxic foods), and the drive to reproduce and care for our young. It is also sometimes described as the primal or reptilian brain, a term coined in the 1980s by the American neuroscientist Paul MacLean, because it controls the self-preserving patterns of behaviour. In anatomy, it is sometimes called the rhinencephalon, which translates literally from the Greek as 'nose-brain'. The link between the olfactory system and the brain lies with the amygdala, the two almond-shaped structures where emotions are given meaning.

Magnetic resonance imaging (MRI) has revealed that when we perceive a scent, the more powerful the memory or emotion associated with the smell, the greater the brain activity. An early study demonstrating this was conducted at Brown University in 2004.[2] Led by Dr Rachel Herz, author of *The Scent of Desire*, one of the first modern books on the psychology of smell, it showed that the brains of women exhibited greater activity when they smelled a perfume they already associated with positive memories than a control fragrance they'd never smelled before.[3] The same effect was produced when they were shown the perfume bottles alone. A more recent study found more brain response when participants were presented with an olfactory stimulus such as the scent of a rose compared with simply looking at the rose.[4] There is continuing important research exploring the powerful role of smells as negative memory triggers for people who have survived violence or trauma and who continue to suffer with post-traumatic stress disorders.

Thomas Hummel is also one of the world's foremost authorities on the effect of anosmia on quality of life and mood and has seen and studied thousands of patients who have either lost their sense of smell or were born without it. He has published extensively on the link between depression and olfactory loss. He is refreshingly matter of fact:

> I always find it funny when you talk to people in the olfactory field because they all say, 'Oh, it is so important', but when we talk to others outside our area and you ask, 'Do we need olfaction?' or you ask them which sense they would lose if they had to choose, people most often opt for olfaction. Olfaction *is* really important but when it comes to people in real life they seem to miss it only when they lose it.

Hummel and his colleagues have conducted extensive research in this area and their findings suggest that depression strikes approximately one third of patients who lose their fifth sense. It is important, he insists, to add a caveat stressing that his subjects are taken from those who attend the clinic – the inference being that they feel the loss intently enough to have sought help. It should be emphasised that smell loss does not always automatically lead to depression: 'Yes, it happens often but not always and when it does occur, for some people it can be severe.' Among patients who have experienced an accompanying phantosmia or parosmia, Hummel says around 35 per cent also exhibit high scores for depression.

The most common changes to quality of life reported by patients in Thomas Hummel's studies relate to the enjoyment of food, with many finding themselves struggling with loss of appetite and consequently eating less. I was heartened to learn that others, although a smaller proportion, were like me and found it hard to feel sated without flavour and therefore found themselves eating more (and gaining weight). A significant but smaller percentage of patients described more difficulties interacting socially, reporting feeling particularly disheartened by the dulling impact on their perception of life in general as well as a dulling of sexual desire.

Thomas Hummel's work shows that while olfactory loss has a major impact on the enjoyment of life and can increase the likelihood of depression, it can also directly affect the functioning of the brain, especially when it comes to emotional control. This is the aspect of recent research that I found most intriguing because it suggests that this lack of sensory input via the olfactory bulb into the limbic system and amygdala might be another pathway to depression.

Studies with laboratory rats who had had their olfactory bulbs surgically removed showed that the lack of odour stimuli to the brain altered serotonin and dopamine levels, the key hormones that stabilise mood. In a study published in 2017, Hummel and his colleague, psychology professor Ilona Croy, revealed that human patients with major depression had significantly smaller olfactory bulbs than age- and sex-matched healthy control patients; this suggests that the *size* of the olfactory bulb could also be an indicator for the severity of mood disease.[5]

The research also showed that otherwise healthy patients born with non-functioning or ill-functioning olfactory bulbs exhibited higher depression scores than the control group. Significantly, studies of patients who reported unhappiness and difficulties growing up revealed their experience had had an impact on the size of the olfactory bulb: 'This effect is also mediated by childhood experience: within a group of depressed patients, those with traumatic childhood experiences exhibit a 20 per cent lower olfactory bulb volume than those patients who report a more or less unremarkable childhood.'

Olfactory bulb volume seems to be related not just to the severity of the depression but also to continuance of the disease. Scans revealed that the depressed patients who had responded well to psychotherapy had significantly higher olfactory bulb volume than those who had shown no improvement over the course of treatment. When the team went back to retest their patients after six months, the volume of their olfactory bulb remained stable. So, not only are patients with olfactory loss more likely to exhibit depressive symptoms but the olfactory bulb itself might constitute an important marker for vulnerability to depression.

＊

A 2015 study compared rats with stress-induced depression with a healthy control group. This revealed that the rats exhibiting depressive behaviours also had a much thinner olfactory epithelium, characterised by fewer receptor neurones.[6] This suggested that if depression slowed the normal turnover of olfactory receptor cells – a process normally controlled by the olfactory bulb – then it might also be worth testing to ascertain whether this growth could be adjusted or encouraged by focusing on the bulb and stimulating it with smells. Professor Hummel's team would show that it's a case of 'use it or lose it': repeated, short-term exposure to smells over a period of twelve weeks significantly improved general olfactory function in their human subjects. This is what we now call smell training. But what is even more interesting, says Professor Hummel, is that further studies have shown that it is possible to target the training and even make it selective, teaching subjects to perceive an odour they barely recognised before.

'Everyone in the world, all of us have some kind of gap or anosmia to some odours. But we know that if you expose people to an odour, you can increase their sensitivity and they can learn to smell it.' An example is androstenone: about one third of the population cannot smell it at all while those who can perceive it as being either similar to sweat or urine and highly unpleasant, or flowery, sweet and rather pleasant.

Professor Hummel says that while the idea that repeated exposure to smells could increase sensitivity had been considered for some time, nobody had tested it in a scientific and clinically controlled way. His earliest work with patients twenty years ago, he recalled, was seen as controversial and greeted with great scepticism by some of his colleagues.

His team persevered and settled on four essential oils chosen from the system of odour classification proposed by the German psychologist Hans Henning in the early twentieth century. Henning's odour prism, published in 1915, placed odours into six primary groups, which he defined as burnt, spicy, resinous, foul, fruity or flowery. Professor Hummel says he chose lemon, eucalyptus, rose and clove, representing the four major pleasant scents, for the training. Over the years, patients have been tested with both single-molecule smells and odour mixtures and the evidence shows now that as long as the smell is strong and the exposure is regular and repetitive over at least three months, there is measurable beneficial effect:

The really interesting thing was that not only did they become more sensitive to the four odours but to many other smells too. A lot of work has been done now to look at the brain and brain function in response to smell training and we have seen that not only is there an increase in the volume of the olfactory bulb but also in the hippocampus and other parts of the brain associated with smell.

We also wanted to see what is happening at the level of the nose and the epithelium, to see if more receptors are being expressed, if it is encouraging regrowth – and there is some evidence that it is.

Professor Hummel says work with electrodes placed inside the nasal cavity has revealed that responses here also increase after smell training but whether this is happening at molecular level and is related to the number of neurones and receptors is a question science has yet to answer.

Is there an area of research that he finds particularly exciting? Professor Hummel doesn't hesitate and describes a research project in which patients learned to recognise the difference between two almost indistinguishable odours, (+)rose oxide and (–)rose oxide.[7] The molecules are mirror images of each other, so you can imagine how similar they smell.

One group received a mild electric shock on their forearm when exposed to one of the rose oxides, but not the other. A control group received no electric shock. When the two groups were tested afterwards, the results revealed that those who received the shock had learned to distinguish between the two smells. This, says Professor Hummel, shows that something is taking place in the nose itself: 'It means that the brain talks to the neurones in the nasal cavity,' he explained. 'That somehow the brain has an effect on the nasal cavity . . . I find this absolutely fascinating.'

As a young postgraduate clinician, Professor Hummel spent time in the United States at the Penn Smell and Taste Center working with its founder, Professor Richard Doty, inventor of the UPSIT (University of Pennsylvania Smell Identification Test), the most widely used self-administered smell test. This is contained in a booklet of forty scratch-and-sniff cards with accompanying multiple-choice questions, which has been used on more than half a million patients since its creation in 1983. Its most recent use with Covid harks back to another pandemic, in the 1930s, when research revealed that monkeys could be protected against the polio virus entering their nasal cavity by damaging their olfactory mucosa – a discovery that would lead to the spraying of children's noses with zinc sulphate as an early protection against polio. The current global epidemic of anosmia, says Professor Hummel, has changed the olfactory research world already: more chemosensory scientists, clinicians and cognitive researchers are working in the field than ever before:

Now, everybody in the population will know somebody who has experienced olfactory loss and, if not, they have at least learned that this can happen, that if you get a respiratory infection you can lose your sense of smell . . . And not only do many more people know that the sense of smell is important and that the consequences of its loss can be pro-found. What is also important is on a political level. Those at the higher levels of government and policy making will have heard the word 'anosmia' and perhaps for the first time will know someone who has had olfactory loss. In the long term, I think this will change the field.

❖

After nearly four decades studying the olfactory system, it remains a source of wonder, mystery and constant surprise to Thomas Hummel. He has recently been studying a young woman who was born congenitally anosmic and whose scans show no visible olfactory bulbs. Yet suddenly, at the age of twenty-four, she has begun to smell. She cannot have a memory of smells because she never experienced or learned them, missing out on all the experiences we undergo as babies and in later childhood that shape our olfactory perception. The shared human response to particular smells and the meaning of the language of smells are alien to her. And yet, says Professor Hummel, this patient exhibits all the precepts of smell shown by people with a standard sense of smell. The clinic had seen her twice at the time of writing and had put her through several batteries of tests, physical and psychological tests along with MRI scans:

> It is fascinating to see. It is all still in its beginning, but her constructs of smell are similar to those of normal people, although she appears to find many odours unpleasant because they are new to her ... these are new experiences that she must become acquainted with. It's a particularly interesting case because she herself is a psychologist. It sounds implausible; it sounds absurd. But in medicine everything is possible ... and it has happened.

18

The Chemistry of Love

Exactly nine months before Covid had begun to wreak its horrors across the globe, the Royal Society, the UK's national academy of sciences, opened the doors of Chicheley Hall, a magnificent early eighteenth-century country house in Buckinghamshire, to an elite group of biologists, psychologists, linguists, anthropologists and chemosensory scientists. The group had come together from all over the world to share the most recent and pioneering research on olfactory communication in humans. More than fifteen papers were presented around the elegant baroque rooms of the villa over the two-day meeting and were published a year later, just as the first reports of anosmia were emerging in the UK.

Delving into what became volume 375, issue 1800, of the Royal Society's *Philosophical Transactions B (Biological)* made me feel like the little anosmic child in Dr Marta Tafalla's novel as she ventured into Baghdad and an Aladdin's cave of olfactory riches. Here were thousands of words describing a dizzying variety of research projects all united by a common belief in the importance of studying the human sense of smell scientifically and systematically.

Christine Drea, Professor of Evolutionary Anthropology at Duke University in Durham, North Carolina, opened proceedings with a paper in which she revealed the potent and varied role of odour in the social lives of a group of primates, particularly the ring-tailed lemur, which goes to inordinate lengths to mix odours, applying scents to its body to influence others and sharing and receiving information about genetic diversity, sexual receptivity and much more through smell.[1] Using examples from 19 other species, Professor Drea explained the evolutionary framework of olfactory behaviour in primates, arguing that the complexity of chemical communication in lemurs can help researchers understand and appreciate the critical role that odorants and chemical communication still play in the social life of humans.

❖

Science continues to show that humans have not lost the neural architecture that allows powerful and sensitive olfactory performance. We might have a smaller olfactory bulb compared with animals we regard as 'super-smellers' such as dogs and mice but we have approximately as many neurones with equal connectivity. While research has shown that dogs and mice respond more sensitively to certain odours, there are many more in which they're matched by humans; at times we can even outperform them. Perhaps one of the most widely quoted early studies highlighting human olfactory performance was conducted in 2006 and published a year later by Berkeley neuroscientists Jess Porter and Noam Sobel who blindfolded and tested thirty-two people to see if they could follow a scent trail of chocolate essence through open grass.[2] Two-thirds of them could – just like sniffer dogs. They then trained four of their subjects three times a day over a twenty-one-day period to see if they improved with practice and they not only followed the trail with greater accuracy but at more than double the speed, instinctively zigzagging their noses backwards and forwards across the odour plume just as dogs do. The study would also shed some light on the way we localise smells, revealing that we do compare scent input to each nostril even though our nostrils are very close together – in a similar way to the way our ears work when we are trying to pinpoint the origin of a sound.

Is it possible then that simple lack of practice, combined with our penchant for deodorising has affected our response to smells? There are areas of life in which we are highly attuned to odour – flowers, perfumes, wines – but these sensitivities are because we sample them often, remind our brains and noses of the varieties of fragrance, the nuances within them. So if our sense of smell is still there, powerful and omnipresent, just how much influence does it have on the way we perceive each other, the mood of a room, another person's interest – or lack of interest? How we choose between prospective partners is one of the most widely studied areas in human olfactory communication. Studies have show, for example, that women rate body odour as more important in mate choice than men.[3]

The scientists in Chicheley Hall during those two spring days in 2019 deemed social olfaction to have 'extraordinary potential' for communication in humans, reporting its powers begin even before we emerge from our mother's womb. The human foetus begins to be able to smell during the last three months of pregnancy. As the baby remains bathed in amniotic fluid, it is permeated by a unique and heady cocktail of odours brewed by the mother's genetic and physiological constitution and seasoned with her dietary choices. Several studies have shown that not only do many food odours scent and flavour amniotic fluid but that newborns will respond physically to the smells they became familiar with or first perceived in utero. This was first shown by a study in which twenty-four newborns were exposed to the unique odour of anise as well as a control smell immediately after birth and again on day four. Infants born to mothers who had consumed anise-spiced food or drinks throughout their pregnancy showed a clear preference for the odour through facial and oral responses while those whose mothers did not ingest anise displayed aversion to it or showed no response.[4]

Anise is a potent flavour and odour, one I would have imagined is an acquired taste that might more commonly come with maturity. The video of the experiment reveals there is no ambiguity about the newborns' faces; their responses confirm vividly that all sorts of tastes from the mother's diet during pregnancy are ingested in utero. This, and other similar studies, suggests that cultural flavours can be experienced and learned well before birth, and mothers can influence the development of their offspring's food preferences in the womb. It also signalled the significant implications involved in early exposure to the odours of addictive substances such as alcohol. Since then, many studies have tested neonates with the odours of an array of other substances, including garlic and ethanol. Newborns exposed to the smell of their own mother's amniotic fluid compared with their reactions to a control odour also reveal a clear preference and head-turning bias, underlining that there is recognition of familiar bodily smells, not just individual compounds.[5]

Maternal smells are clearly central to the life of a developing infant, guiding the most important post-natal behaviours. I wonder why the role of the olfactory system is not more widely known, taught to young mothers as part of pre-natal preparation. From latching onto the breast in the hours following birth to the development of healthy eating and drinking habits to a continuing role in the cementing of the relationship between parent and child, smells and olfactory experience seems to prepare the groundwork for each life stage as it unfolds.

German scientists attending the Royal Society meeting revealed that over and beyond that first potent, bonding whiff, maternal – indeed parental – olfactory responses continue to play a significant and extraordinary role not only in promoting parental care but also in protection of the species. They showed that the nose can also behave like a sentinel, ensuring mothers can recognise their biological child's body odour (preferring the smell of their own child to that of others, including stepchildren) which promotes targeted parental care. And later in life, we find much more attractive the body odour of those who do not share similarities in the human leukocyte antigen system, the gene complex that encodes important elements of our immune system.

If this finding isn't extraordinary enough, the same German researchers told the Royal Society meeting that over the course of childhood, parental perception of their child's body odours appears to change and the smell of children of the opposite sex is perceived as less pleasant in puberty, suggesting some chemosensory protections and innate smell aversion against inbreeding. The stench of a teenager's bedroom, it seems, could have an evolutionary foundation.

19

Smell is the Scaffolding

Charles Darwin, elected to the Royal Society aged just thirty, was the first to foresee that scent probably drives the neonate human's inexorable journey towards their mother's nipple. The naturalist kept a private diary in 1840 in which he observed his newborn son's behaviours, from birth to toddlerhood. Darwin would return to these detailed notes some thirty-seven years later, using them as a basis of a paper titled 'A biographical sketch of an infant' published in the journal *Mind* in 1877. 'I had excellent opportunities for close observation and wrote down at once whatever was observed,' he wrote cheerily, both scientist and doting father.[1] It would take science another hundred years to corroborate Darwin's hunch.

Despite its extraordinary importance to the survival of human babies, olfactory perception in newborns was largely ignored by researchers until the mid 1970s when a couple of laboratories in Europe and the United States turned their attention in earnest to trying to pinpoint exactly what drives a newborn to the breast. The first and most important of these studies was undertaken in 1975 and revealed that seventeen out of twenty breastfed neonates aged two to seven days immediately recognise and turn towards their mother's smell.[2] Later experiments would reveal that even bottle-fed babies turn towards – and prefer – the breast odour of an unfamiliar lactating woman over their familiar formula milk or even the axillary (armpit) odour of their own mother.[3] This suggested to scientists that the scent emitted from the breast – but perhaps not breast milk itself – could be a fundamental driver of baby's earliest behaviours.

Could it be that the breast itself plays a role as a scent organ? This was suggested by several different studies that documented newborns' directional crawl to the breast when placed prone on the mother's torso within an hour of birth or when placed on a mattress and presented with a scentless pad compared to a pad impregnated with their mother's breast (not milk) odour.[4]

This has been observed countless times but why it occurs and what substance drives it remains a mystery although there are increasingly persuasive theories that those little, seemingly useless bumps that surround the nipple on the areola may well be the source of the scent that is so irresistible to tiny babies. Studies have shown that the more of these little bumps the women have, the quicker their milk comes in – and the faster their babies put on weight. The bumps also secrete a substance to which babies are drawn. This effect was greater in first-time mothers who began lactating an average of ten hours earlier than those with fewer glands – and their babies fed more frequently too. Dr Benoist Schaal observed that it appeared that the breast-feeding relationship appeared to be more difficult for first-time mothers with lower numbers of areolar glands: 'Babies of first-time mothers may then be more reliant on olfactory cues as their mothers are less familiar with other signals that their infant wants to feed.'[5]

The odour produced by what are known as Montgomerian secretions have since become the subject of many more studies because it seems that while babies appear to be attracted in a similar way by the scent of their mother's whole breast as well as the isolated areola, nipple and drops of milk, they show a very different kind of excitement when presented with the odour of the secretions produced by the bumps, breathing more quickly and with a more frenzied suckling response.[6]

The more I learned, the more I wondered how it is possible that modern chemosensory science has discovered so much about the importance of smell in foetal and infant development and yet nothing is taught to children or parents – or general practitioners – to make us more aware of its role in holistic health. Just as powerful is the significance and implication of these studies in paediatrics, particularly as modern medicine has found ways to save the lives of more and more pre-term babies when finding ways to stimulate feeding after long periods of naso-gastric feeding in incubators is imperative.

Dr Schaal, now one of the world's leading researchers on olfaction in early childhood, had delivered an important paper to the Royal Society meeting that outlined the leaps and bounds made by science in documenting the importance of the sense of smell as a scaffold for learning from in utero to toddlerhood and adolescence – work that has been described as 'critical'. In an email exchange about the meeting, Professor Craig Roberts described Dr Schaal's discoveries on the human areola as scent organs as one of 'his favourite papers of all time'. Professor Roberts suggested I interview more scientists involved in this kind of research in an effort to make it more widely known. Serendipity struck not very long after we chatted: the opportunity arose to meet Dr Schaal at Professor Thomas Hummel's six-day Summer School on Olfaction in Dresden, Germany. European travel bans lifted just in time for me to accept the invitation.

As I prepped on the plane, the list of lecturers made me feel as if I'd be meeting the rock stars of the smell world, a collection of the top medics and scientists working at the very cutting edge of smell research in Europe and the US. These were the women and men whose peer-reviewed papers I had been reading for more than a year but now I would be able to put faces to names, talk to them, ask questions in person.

Dr Schaal turned out to be a tall man with a thick mop of hair, slightly dishevelled in the way of the scientist who has been forced out of the lab and into a collared shirt and tailored trousers for a special occasion. He speaks a perfect, joyously French-accented English and during a lecture that lasted two and a half hours, ranged eloquently over three decades of research, illustrating the detail of experiments conducted with babies less than three days old, showing video of their faces screwed up in disgust at some scents (lemon, fishy or rotten egg) and smiling openly at the ones they recognised (milk, colostrum) or others they appeared to deem innately pleasant (vanilla, butter).

As a zoologist and animal-behaviour specialist, he talked about his team's research with mammals and primates and enthralled the lecture theatre with the results of several years of studies on newborn rabbit pups – more than 7,000 of them were tested – which ultimately revealed that of the dozens of molecular compounds in the rabbit mother's milk, just one component, identified as 2-methyl-but-2-enal (aka 2MB2) was as powerful as whole milk in eliciting the rabbit pup's frenzied grasping and rooting for the smell offered from a tiny glass pipette.

Painstaking work with GC-O saw the researchers literally pull the milk apart into its many separate molecular compounds, which were then presented individually to the rabbit babies to observe their responses. It took years but Schaal's team was able to identify a true 'mammary pheromone', chemicals produced by an animal that by itself influences the behaviour of an individual of the same species.[7] Of the thousands of rabbit pups tested, around 10 per cent did not react to the pheromone at all and this non-reactive cohort all failed to survive to weaning. This underlined the importance of this particular odour to survival of the rabbit species:

> 2MB2 is not found in amniotic fluid, nor in blood so we were able to rule out pre-natal learning. It is an olfactory signal, a single compound at fixed ratio and has specific receptivity. It does not work with any other animal, no others reacted and didn't work with human babies either. We have been working long and working hard with humans but we haven't found anything like it.

One of the most extraordinary pieces of study footage Schaal showed us was the frenzy induced by the substance when it was piped to a large group of rabbit babies who had been sleeping in big, warm, languorous heaps. Within seconds they were awake – eyes not yet open after birth – desperately rolling and squirming, walking over each other, scratching blindly to try to find the source of the delectable smell. And yet this dramatic response begins to disappear after the tenth day after birth when the pups begin to open their eyes in preparation for solid food sources and researchers realised its seemingly magical power has completely disappeared by thirty days – the usual time rabbit females wean their babies.

The same substance was also detected in the rabbit mother's anus, showing that she was transmitting the odour to her faecal pellets, later attracting her babies to ingest them and help adapt their intestinal microbiota to the grasses and herbs they would encounter in the big wide world outside. For the rabbit, the 2MB2 is a fundamental plank in what scientists call ontogenetic adaptation, the process of distinct and co-ordinated steps and stages of learning that prepare infant animals to survive in the external environment away from their parents.

If anyone needed any further proof of the power of odour over vision in these earliest moments in a human baby's life, Dr Schaal referred us to a series of experiments conducted with his colleague Sébastien Doucet in which three- and four-day-old babies were presented with their mother's breast over two consecutive trials:

One was with the breast entirely covered in transparent, plastic film so it was visible to the babies but scentless. This was paired with four conditions, one with a fully exposed breast, one with only the nipple exposed, one with the areola alone and the other with milk available.

The babies that could see but not smell the breast cried earlier and for longer and opened their eyes less but were more orally activated when they were exposed to nipple, areola and milk odours which all delayed crying onset.[8]

Seeing their mother's breast simply isn't enough for human babies. And just to cement these finds, another study with older infants aged around four months tracked their eye movements electronically as they were shown still pictures of a car and a female face.[9] As expected, they focused much more on the face but when they were shown it in the presence of their mother's odour, the baby's spontaneous preference was pronounced and they looked longer at the eyes than any other facial parts. 'Maternal odour boosts engagement of vision and may also help promote rapid recognition of faces, vision-based reward systems, empathy and the onset of attachment, bonding and the liberation of oxytocin [the hormone involved in social bonding],' Dr Schaal said.

We humans often alter our odour with scents and fragrances – who doesn't remember their mother's favourite perfume in early childhood? And yet, human babies have been shown to learn even these synthetic smells very quickly, recognising their familiarity and offering clearly happy facial responses even in their mother's absence.

20

The Smell of Fear

While most olfactory scientists are students of the human brain, nose and smell-driven behaviours, Professor Jonathan Williams, an atmospheric chemist at the Max Planck Institute in Germany, studies air. The connection between atmospheric chemistry and the sense of smell may seem a little indirect and deserves explanation: when odour molecules are released into the air, let's say from a fruit ripening on a vine, the initial concentration of the smell diminishes over time and fades away with distance from the source. This is not just because odour molecules become diluted into the surrounding air but also because sunlight breaks them down in a process known as photo-oxidation.

Human noses don't detect all smells equally. The ones we are most sensitive to are compounds found in nature. Some of these can be detected at extremely low concentration while others we barely perceive at all. Williams and his colleague Akima Ringsdorf told the Royal Society that they now think they know why. They compared the contents of a smell sensitivity database, compiled over more than a decade by Japanese scientists, with an atmospheric chemistry database. This meant they could compare the smell thresholds with the lifespan of an array of organic molecules in the air. Their findings revealed a striking link between chemical families such as alcohols and esters associated with some foods, particularly fruits, and nitrogen and sulphur compounds associated with fire and bodily wastes.

Evolution and adaptation, they suggest, has led us to become most responsive to the chemicals that react most quickly with other elements in the air and then disintegrate and disappear just as quickly from our noses. These are specialised olfactory sensitivities that help us find – and quickly identify – danger or toxic substances. Williams told colleagues at the Royal Society conference:

> A good sense of smell is a big advantage when looking for food. If you want to find a nutritious ripe fruit in a dense, dark forest you need to be able to follow a smell gradient as it twists and turns in turbulent air streams. And the molecules with the shortest lifetimes have the steepest gradients. The results we have seem to support the general hypothesis that there is a link between atmospheric chemistry and the sense of smell, which nobody had thought of before.

●

Williams came into the field of human smell by accident. He has spent more than two decades researching how gases emitted into the Earth's atmosphere contribute to climate change and embarks on a twice-yearly odyssey involving large and small aircraft, cars and a final climb on foot to work in a 325-metre-high research tower built deep in the Amazon by his institute. Here, he and his research assistants and students use a suite of sensitive instruments to measure how specific gases emitted into the air by vegetation (volatile organic compounds) react in the air and contribute to the production of ozone and other particles.

In 2016, a member of his student group, driven by sheer curiosity, decided to blow into one of the highly sensitive instruments designed to capture the fresh forest air and, to the team's surprise, the breath sample was found to contain a similar array of the substances released by Amazonian jungle plants, including lots of isoprene, one of its major constituents. This raised the question: could it be that we humans, all 7.5 billion of us, are contributing to climate change?

Williams returned to Germany determined to try to interrogate the possibility that human breath could be an ingredient in global warming and, as a classic football-fan scientist, decided he would test his idea by taking measurements of the air above a 31,000-seat football stadium. These would show that when something exciting happened in the match or anxiety and frustration were running high, levels of similar organic compounds in the air rose. Further studies conducted in a cinema during a range of different films seemed to confirm that the fluctuations were related to human emotion and that tension and even relief can literally be read in the air (something that anosmics would not be aware of). When pulses rise and people become tense in their seats as a suspenseful moment unfolds on the screen, the levels of carbon dioxide and isoprene rise, the latter seemingly stored in the muscle tissue as the audience tenses.

But what about other feelings? Could sadness, affection, arousal also be measured in the air? Williams and his team turned next to breaking responses down by movie type, turning to data specialists who normally analyse economic fluctuations. They found that the most obvious link emerged with suspenseful scenes followed by comedy and laughter, perhaps revealing an evolutionary advantage because 'alert' or 'stand-down' signals are so important for survival.[1] If these chemical changes can be detected in the air by instruments, is it possible that our noses are registering them too, and that, without consciously knowing it, we really can smell fear?

The expression and reading of fear in humans has fascinated psychologists and neuroscientists for decades, although research has focused primarily on examining axillary (armpit) sweat and facial expressions as participants are exposed to an array of stimuli, from aggression and violence during video games to the effects of watching winners and losers in martial arts contests. Previous studies[2] have revealed that a person experiencing fear or terror emits sweat[3] that is measurably different at molecular level to that of a person who is neutral or happy and that the production of these fear odours engages the same areas of the brain used to process frightened and fearful facial expressions. But while much work has been done to show that humans can decode this emotional intensity in each other's faces, nobody had yet tried yet to see if this is also true of olfaction.

Jasper de Groot, an assistant professor at Radboud University in the Netherlands, was fascinated by the idea and started to investigate. He and his collaborators began testing their hypothesis on fear odours and intensity by collecting fear and neutral sweat from pads placed under the armpits of thirty-six participants as they watched half-hour movie clips using horror to elicit fear and gentle nature documentaries to induce calm. The scientists then measured their subjective responses along with physiological markers such as heart rate and ranked them into three groups: those who, when watching horror films, experienced low, medium and high amounts of fear. Those who exhibited most fear not only sweated more but also emitted a higher quantity of volatile odorant molecules.

The 'receiver' group was female as women tend to have more sensitive noses and, according to the authors, are more likely to respond emotionally and less consciously to smell cues. An olfactometer, specially equipped to deliver air in a natural way as if through clothing or straight from the body, delivered the four categories of odours – neutral, low, medium and high fear – and participants were asked to rate both the pleasantness and intensity. However, before the odour was delivered, they were shown images of two male actors who had been photographed showing fearful or disgusted faces but were Photoshopped to create more ambiguous, difficult-to-read facial expressions. The female 'reader' group was asked to choose if the face was showing fear or disgust.

The results were a surprise. Instead of perceiving more fear in the ambiguous faces when exposed to sweat from the high-fear groups, the receivers could not distinguish between them, effectively reading fear in all the faces. When the effects of the different doses of fear sweat were examined at physiological and neural level, these also activated the parts of the brain linked to fight and flight or fear. So, even at minute doses, each level of fear sweat transmitted by a sender was perceived and processed very quickly by the receiver.

The scientists elegantly described their findings as a 'temporal winner-takes-all principle', one that suggests that we're sensitively wired to smell fear at all levels because, let's face it, it's always better to be safe than sorry.

21

Speaking of Smells

I had never really thought about this before I lost my sense of smell but think it fair to say that while many animals communicate their reactions to stimuli in different ways, it is only humans who can articulate the subtleties of our sensations and how they make us feel. We share the joy of a hug from a child or lover, describe the breath-snatching beauty of the colours of a sunset, reminisce about being covered in goose bumps while listening to Bach's *St Matthew Passion* in an ancient, stone cathedral. But why is it that we find it so difficult to describe smells, to find words that encapsulate a transporting fragrance (or a vile stench) without resorting to the source of the odour? What do sun-kissed, ripe strawberries smell like? Well, um, like ripe strawberries.

Some experts put this down to a lack of descriptors or adjectives in Indo-European languages, arguing that we would describe them better if only we had more words for them. One very recent study concluded that the English language has fewer smell-associated words than words for any other sense and that of 40,000 words chosen to represent a full adult vocabulary, 74 per cent were deemed to be vision-dominated while less than one per cent related to smell.[1] Another data-crunching exercise took 8 million words from 7,000 British English texts containing first-person descriptions of the splendours of the Lake District and of these, nearly 29,000 related to sight, around 1,500 to sound – and just 78 referred to smell.[2,3]

Odour, argue some researchers, is ineffable – almost impossible to put into words. Others, like *What the Nose Knows* author and sensory psychologist Avery Gilbert, disagree, insisting that almost every smelly thing in the world can be a potential adjective or descriptor – lemons, oranges, onion, petrol – not to mention the vast array of brands known for their recognisable scents, from Vicks VapoRub and Play-Doh to Texta permanent markers or the indelible British antiseptic TCP. In the view of researchers such as Gilbert, it's not the lack of vocabulary but an issue of cognition: the words are there but we have a hard time pulling them up, foiled by what he calls the 'verbal barrier'. Professor Barry Smith described smell as the 'orphan' sense, one that requires all the other senses to help it work and to work with it, highlighting the difficulty most people encounter identifying even familiar smells when blindfolded.

This so-called 'tip of the nose' syndrome was first described by the Norwegian sensory psychologist the late Trygg Engen in 1977 during a series of experiments in which he investigated these very common and yet strong feelings of imminent recall about odour identification. His team asked participants to sniff and identify a selection of forty-eight odours but if they were unable to name one but still deemed it familiar, they were offered a series of further, semantic clues. In seven out of ten cases, given the extra information, they were able to pinpoint the smell.

Later studies have also shown that this feeling of knowing a smell is indeed a good predictor that participants will later identify it correctly.[4]

However, when asked to identify sets of common odours such as tar, coffee and cinnamon, people rarely score above 50 per cent – and compared with images, smells take up to four times longer to name. This fits exactly with what I had discovered first-hand in Dr Jane Parker's laboratory and the sniffing pens: that more often than not I knew the smell – chocolate, coffee, strawberry, banana – but no matter how hard I tried, without any context I just couldn't put my finger (or nose) on its name.

When we read or hear language that involves vision or hearing, areas of the brain that are involved in both perception and action light up. In 2007, researchers at University College London tested the impact of language on the senses, asking subjects to listen to verbs related to an upward or downward movement and to perform an associated task. The experiment revealed that when the verb spoken was incongruent with the movement the subjects were seeing, they hesitated, delayed their verbal response, and both their perception and performance of the movement was impaired.[5] It seems that we don't just see or hear or think about these senses in an abstract way alone. Our brains try to grasp a way to recreate or 'embody' the experience and make it 'real'.

Yet with smell and taste we don't seem to have that same, quick link with language. There have been myriad theories to explain this gap, some arguing that odour perception is multi-modal and so needs context and interaction with the other senses, making it much more difficult to conjure up and imagine in isolation, while others suggest limits of connectivity between language and olfactory areas of the brain. Still others propose that because odours are rarely spoken about in detail, children have little opportunity to learn to talk about smells.[6] There is also no real agreement within the scientific community about whether the connection between olfaction and language is symmetrical or asymmetrical, in other words whether it is as difficult to conjure smells from words as it is to find a word to describe a smell.

Close your eyes for a moment and imagine that a government decree has been issued that makes the word 'green' illegal. Could you find a way to describe the colour? Would you choose to use 'tree', 'meadow', 'a cat's eyes'? How do you describe the group or category of 'green' things without mentioning the 'g' word? That is the issue for us Europeans, English speakers and most others: we simply don't have categories to describe groups or families of smells.

Psychology Professor Asifa Majid, a cognitive scientist and linguist at the University of York, is at the forefront of research on olfactory language and has documented and written extensively about cultures and communities that share a far richer smell lexicon than we have.[7] Her work with Huehuetla Tepehua, the language spoken by an indigenous group of peoples in the Sierra Madre Mountains of north-eastern Mexico, has revealed that not only do they have wide categories to describe families of smells but also use ideophones – similar to onomatopoeic words that evoke a noise such as *bang!* or *achoo!* – to deliver a sense of intensity. For example, vowels delivered at a high pitch or consonants made at the front of the mouth evoke a nuanced, less intense perception of a smell than a low-pitched sound produced at the back of the mouth.

Smell can be a source of metaphor in English, but more often than not, according to Majid's work, these contain negatives ('this situation stinks'), suspicion ('I smell a rat') or searching and investigation ('they're sniffing for clues'). And yet there are other cultures where smell is used fluidly as metaphor: in Luwo, a language of Sudan, it is used in reference, for example, to aspects of knowledge. Seri, the language of a hunter-gatherer group in Mexico is enlivened by an elaborate smell vocabulary that includes olfactory metaphors used to describe emotions.

Majid decided to go out into the field to see if the struggle faced by English speakers to name the things they smell is universally true across other languages and cultures.[8] She led a team of twenty-six scientists who fanned out all over the globe and, using the same set of colours, shapes, sounds, tactile textures, tastes and odours, put the question to the test. The researchers had imagined that if a single, universal hierarchy of the senses exists, the peoples studied would communicate best and most easily about vision, followed by sound, textures, taste and, finally, smell.

The team discovered that it is not biology but culture that predicts the relative importance of the senses. Speakers of Farsi and Lao, for example, communicated with great ease about basic tastes, something that English speakers found much harder and that the researchers suggested could be a result of differences in how people engaged with their cultural cuisine. In Kata Kolok, a sign language used in Bali, Indonesia, researchers found both signs and facial expressions that eloquently communicated sweet and sour tastes, while Siwu speakers in Ghana excelled at describing textures, perhaps thanks to a lively culture of handiwork and food preparation. Cultures that produced intricate and patterned pottery used language abundant with adjectives and words referring to shapes, while cultures that valued specialist musical heritage were the most efficient describing sounds. Yet, despite these myriad variations among cultures, the study concluded with the caveat that smell is still poorly communicated uniformly across the board: most human beings need to resort to the source for description because a strawberry smells like, well, a strawberry.

※

Modern olfactory science is very much dominated by research focused on receptors and understanding the molecular basis of how and why we smell what we do. However, there is also a growing body of research voices who argue the need to widen the lens through which memory and the use of language shapes human perception of odours. Majid, like Professor Craig Roberts and his colleagues, believes that researchers must turn to more non-Western groups in their studies and a cross-cultural approach is imperative if we are to understand how humans communicate about smells. It was her lab's study of the Jahai-speaking Semaq Beri I mentioned to illustrate a group for whom smell sits front and centre of both cultural and linguistic practices.[9]

Majid's work there revealed that using three different measures, the Jahai speakers were more consistent and successful naming smells over colours than control participants tested in the Netherlands. 'Our findings show that these long-held assumptions that people are bad at naming smells is not universally true,' she wrote. 'Odours are expressible in language, as long as you speak the right language.' For example, one word can describe an abstract, broad category of smells and in Jahai *cŋɛs* (pronounced something like 'chnges') encapsulates the smell of smoke and petrol, the stench of bat droppings and bat caves, some types of millipedes, the root of wild ginger and the wood of wild mango among other odour sources.

More recently, in a research paper simply titled 'Hunter Gatherer Olfaction is Special', Majid and her linguist colleague Nicole Kruspe compare the Semaq Beri with the neighbouring Semelai who are not foragers but use slash-and-burn agricultural techniques, cultivate rice and trade foraged forest foods to survive.[10] The Maniq and Jahai people live in the fecund valleys around the Tembeling river in Malaysia's Taman Negara National Park, speak similar languages and share similar physical characteristics, including short stature and peppercorn hair.

The researchers specially selected a series of odours captured in Professor Thomas Hummel's Sniffin' Sticks along with swatches of colours. They then categorised the responses into those who agreed on how to describe a smell, whether they chose a source-based word such as 'banana' or 'fish', whether they rated it for its pleasantness or intensity, and if they used an abstract description. There was no control condition; the researchers simply calculated agreement, coding responses into 'good', 'bad' or abstract. The results were both intriguing and unexpectedly stark in their differences because the hunter-gatherer Semaq Beri used many more particular, abstract terms to describe groups of odours or their qualities, while the farming Semelai found it much more difficult to name smells than they did colours, generally replicating the findings among the more well-studied Western psychology undergraduates.

This suggests that language can very much influence not only how accurately you can label a mystery smell but also on how likely it is that you will agree with others about what that mystery smell is. Kruspe, who completed her PhD in Australia, told the *New York Times* that she had expected the differences between the two groups to be much more subtle although the importance a cultural group places on odour obviously has a major influence on how it is valued and described. Of course, it makes complete sense that communities that rely on the natural environment, on the forests and its plants and animals to survive will build spiritual and kinship practices around smell and prioritise the sensory information that not only helps to identify food but can also warn against danger. The question for researchers now is just how long these olfactory practices can survive against the relentless advance of the modern, deodorising world – and if the generations that come after will manage to retain these skills.

So why do humans have such difficulties translating our experience from the nose to the word? The conundrum spurred another neuroscientist colleague, Artin Arshamian, to join forces with Majid to seek some answers. Their interesting and novel theory argues that we find it particularly hard to label the things we smell compared with the things we hear or see because olfactory imagery – the process that allows us to close our eyes and imagine a banana or conjure up its shape and colour in the mind's eye – does not pass through the same process of 'embodiment' that helps us learn to decipher the world through the other senses.[11] As children, we see new things, touch and play with them, put them in our mouth to get a true feel of them. And whether we are aware of it or not, as adults our bodies are always working for us and acting as the touchstone for our senses. At times, says Majid, we even use parts of our bodies to explain wider concepts both in space and relating to emotions. For example, the word 'face' refers to a part of our head but we also use the word to locate something, for example, 'My house faces the park.' The same word can communicate a change of mind: 'He did an about-face.' Or communicate the fear of embarrassment: 'She didn't want to lose face.'

Most of the information we perceive is of course provided to us by our bodies: shapes, colours, textures, temperatures, tastes and smells. Many theories about how we learn to recognise objects and add to our repertoire of knowledge suggest that we match what we see against simple structural representations of objects in the brain. Psychologists call these 'geons', groups of two- or three-dimensional forms such as spheres, cubes, cylinders, cones and wedges that, when broken down, can be recombined into an innumerable number of other forms. An ice-cream cone, for example, can be deconstructed into a cone and a sphere and some theorists have proposed that just twenty-four geons can be recombined to create more than 10 million different two-geon objects.

Arshamian and Majid argue that with smell there is no such direct link between an 'image' and the body so there are far fewer opportunities to train ourselves to build these essential mental pictures. In utero, a foetus is a passive recipient of stimuli to all its senses but in infancy children begin to experiment actively and produce sounds, mimic facial expressions, practise and consolidate responses to the things their senses perceive, the things they can see, hear and touch. And they continue to practise and reproduce these responses as they mature and grow. But with smell, opportunities to manipulate the odour stimuli are limited and the ability to 'embody' or visualise them is almost impossible.

As I absorbed the researchers' paper in order to write about it, I realised that even in the description of my own 'tip of the nose' experience, I'd used another part of the body – 'I can't put my finger on it' – to explain the inability to grasp what I was smelling. It seemed to make so much sense that olfactory representations and imagery within our imagination simply cannot have the same solidity because we have so much less opportunity to learn how to do it over our lifetimes. Work examining this with Dutch adults and children aged nine to twelve confirmed that while the sharpness of visual and auditory images often develops and becomes even more vivid with age, the same simply doesn't happen with smell 'images'.

Majid and her colleagues point out that while studies examining the ability to conjure olfactory imagery suggests that it is difficult to relate findings across cultures, nobody has embarked on targeted studies of hunter-gatherer communities for comparison. She observed:

It is possible that in [these] communities, the use, interaction and embodiment of odours in everyday life shapes olfactory cognition deeply, even at representational level. For example, the fact that some cultures monitor and

manipulate odours to avert sickness suggests a level of conscious awareness beyond what is displayed by lay people in
the West. Similarly, we saw that many communities have
developed lexicons for smells emitted by different parts of
the body. If this is something children are being encultured
into early in life, perhaps it deepens the embodiment.

The reality is that there is still no real agreement between scientists and philosophers about the hows and whys of our poor
olfactory language, including the idea that we put smells together
in the same way we 'understand' facial characteristics. This was
tested by two Australian researchers, Stevenson and Mahmut,
who set up a set of clever and rather complex experiments at
Macquarie University in Sydney using thirty smells matched to
pictures and distracting images.[12] Their work illustrated that even
when we can't identify a face – and we're not that great at remembering unfamiliar faces anyway – we still have access to words or
semantic cues about the face: big nose, small eyes, high cheek-
bones. These elements help us build an informational picture
as a whole. But if we are given odorants to smell, it's incredibly
difficult to find associated, semantic information to help. This
suggests there is poor connectivity between our olfactory perceptual centres (the orbital frontal cortex) and those that process our
language memories (primarily the dorsomedial and ventromedial
frontal cortex). In other words, they argue that we suffer from a
connectivity shortfall.

Our poor accuracy at identifying odours cannot be explained
away by the notion that we are no good at smelling: we now
know the opposite is true for humans despite centuries of

underestimating our skills. And while we don't have a definitive answer to explain the discrepancy, we do know olfactory language is built by experience and learning working hand in hand – and that this process might even shape our perception of smell itself.

22

Parfum Eau de Poo

The strangest thing about becoming anosmic after Covid – as thousands of people around the world attest daily on social media – is that if you are lucky and begin to recover, the path is unpredictable and sometimes deeply frustrating.

Sixteen months after infection, my sense of smell had returned to the point that I felt both a daily, heart-singing gratitude and a sense of relief I couldn't measure. Every morning, the ritual sniffing of my collection of perfumes as part of the suggested retraining regime turned into tiny instants of celebration as familiar scents I feared were gone for ever returned and began at last to match my memory of them.

I always began my sniffing-fest by uncapping an anti-frizz hair product my sister-in-law Karen had given to me during my last visit to Australia, just before the pandemic began. It is made from the oil of the prickly pear cactus and I loved it for its texture and a barely perceptible, honeyed and yet clearly vegetal fragrance. When I opened the bottle to massage a few drops into my hands and then onto my hair, it transported me instantly to those long afternoons at the beach, showering at my mum's place and the humid heat of a Sydney summer. But for months, it was a ghost, there in golden liquid form before my eyes but undetectable to my Covid-seared epithelium. When this one returned, the relief was overwhelming because I knew that it offers a vague scent, one you had to concentrate on. The minute it came back, it flooded me with happy memories.

Similarly, I cannot forget the excitement of my favourite perfume rematerialising into a head full of the rich, smoky, leather-musk scent I'd happily bathe in (if it weren't so expensive). The day I began to perceive it again is marked in my diary with a phalanx of red hearts as if I were a lovelorn teenager. I used to spritz myself with this fragrance every day and it permeated my watch strap and sweaters, foofing out in an invisible plume when I opened my drawers or wardrobe door. It had been a Christmas gift from Robert and our youngest daughter says she now equates it with me. (For the record, Le Labo's Santal 33 has notes of an exotic mix of Australian sandalwood, cardamom, leather accord, iris and ambrox, which in my mind is equal parts spice and smoke).

Of all these moments, the most inexplicable lay with my bizarre perception of a cheap but still rather lovely Body Shop jasmine oil that I'd often dab on in midwinter simply to evoke the feeling of spring. In the early days of recovery, that was the only perfume that didn't smell vague but stank in a way I can barely describe: a rancid mix of chemical, metallic but putrid faeces, as if every ingredient in the little bottle had been left in the sun to stew and warp. It was so awful that I became convinced it had changed colour and gone off and I'd have thrown it away if it weren't for the network of parosmia sufferers who kept posting on AbScent's Facebook pages to describe the weird and wild things they too were experiencing. Curious, I decided to hang on to it and kept sniffing this one religiously along with my other perfumes. Then one day, out of the blue – just before I set off to Dresden for Professor Hummel's Olfactory Summer School – the little bottle smelled of a jasmine bush in full flower again. It was as if some kind of mysterious process had occurred in the glass but by then I had learned that the answer to the riddle lay with my olfactory system and smell receptors regenerating – not the contents of the bottle. I still smell it every day without fail, feeling relief every single time I inhale its rich, floral scent.

*

Dr Christian Margot, a Swiss chemist based in Geneva, had travelled to Dresden to give a lecture on molecular chemistry. I had been immediately interested in what he might say because while all the other lecturers had sent scientific papers for us to read in preparation, Dr Margot had sent only a short tract of text from Franz Kafka's 1926 novel *The Castle* along with some questions for us to ponder. Dark and often surreal, the story is narrated by a protagonist known only as 'K', its dystopian feel particularly stark when you know Kafka died of tuberculosis before he could finish it. I read and re-read the two paragraphs Dr Margot had sent us during the bus journey between Berlin and Dresden as rain pelted the windows and dark clouds scudded by as we travelled the autobahn. I could not help but wonder what would link the fragrance scientist's work with the German-speaking, Bohemian modernist writer.

When he entered the lecture room, to our surprise Dr Margot was carrying a bottle of cognac with his laptop and proceeded to pour a nip for each of us into tiny, disposable cups. We settled into our seats with the fragrant amber liquid in front of us under orders that, for now, we must sniff only and not taste or drink as he read a short tract of Kafka's text. For context, we knew that it was deep winter and protagonist K is wrapped up in a rug in a horse-drawn sleigh, warm and sheltered from the snow when his coachman offers him a cognac while he runs an errand:

> Clumsily, without altering his position, he reached across the side pocket, not in the open door, which was too distant, but behind him in the closed one, after all it did not matter, there were bottles inside this pocket too. He pulled one out, unscrewed the cap and took a sniff, instinctively he had to smile, the smell was so sweet, caressing and as delightful as hearing praise and kind words from someone you love but you don't know why, nor do you want to know, you are just happy to hear the beloved person uttering them. 'Can this really be cognac?' K. wondered, tasting it out of curiosity. Yes, it was cognac, remarkably enough, burning and warming him. But as he drank it, it turned from something that was little more than the vehicle for sweet perfumes into a drink more suitable for a coach driver. 'Is it possible?' wondered K. as if in need of proof and took another sip.

As we sniffed our own tiny glasses of the distilled wine, everybody had a similar experience, the fragrance offering a honey-like effect, golden, soothing and overwhelmingly described as 'sweet' – even though that is a taste descriptor. And yet once we had it on the tongue, it bit us like it bit K, stimulating the trigeminal nerve and producing a mix of bitterness and heat a world away from the scent. I'm not sure I had ever even tasted a good cognac before let alone spent a couple of hours smelling it but by the time Dr Margot's lecture was over, the chasm between K's perception of the smell of cognac versus the in-mouth experience was much clearer.

While scientists believe that the variety of food smells is almost unlimited, the vast majority are created by a combination of around 230 key odorants. However, the heady fragrance of cognac, distilled and then aged in wood, has been shown to consist of 500 different molecules with most attributable to a group of thirty-six, including carbon, hydrogen, nitrogen, oxygen and sulphur along with thiol, which, Dr Margot told us, has a sulphur atom in the place of oxygen. One, 4-mercapto-4-methylpentan-2-one, or 4MMP, has the more user-friendly name of the 'cat ketone'. This is the one that some people perceive as slightly urine-like in Sauvignon Blanc. (I have been known to send my Sauvignon Blanc-loving mother into a paroxysm when I have described her favoured New Zealand tipple as smelling like 'cat piss'.)

Dr Margot asked us to think about cognac's smell structure as a little like a sculpture constructed of Lego: with so many unique molecules involved, it is inordinately difficult to work out or predict what to put into the barrels to attain particular scents and flavours. 'This is so difficult because, like so many things with smell, we don't actually understand it,' he said.

The nose-versus-mouth experience described by K in Kafka's novel allowed him to provide a poetic illustration of the way orthonasal olfaction – the act of pure sniffing – offers an entirely different experience from retronasal olfaction, which unfolds when we chew or swallow, ensuring odour molecules bounce around the tongue and mouth, wafting up behind the uvula and then up into the nasal cavity to reach the olfactory epithelium. Dr Margot paced the floor, saying:

I asked you to think about why it elicits a smile in K. This is because he loves the smell, because he has an emotion as he smells it . . . it's not about the wood and the spice and the tingling from vanilla and all that stuff you hear from wine connoisseurs. K smiles because he has an emotional reaction, it is that first immediate response, that like or dislike. And yet when he tastes it, it is nothing like the smell. It is not sweet, it is hidden beneath bitterness. Again, these are emotional words depending on the emotional experience.

Identifying the links between smell and emotion has been Dr Margot's bread and butter for decades, leading multi-disciplinary teams from academic institutions with perfumers and olfactory researchers, chemists and psychologists, to deepen understanding of how our sense of smell interacts with our sentiments. He is Director of Human Perception and Bioresponses at Firmenich, the world's biggest private company working in the fragrance and flavours business. Founded in 1900 as a perfumery, Firmenich later branched into flavours, launching the first raspberry substitute in 1938 followed quickly by man-made citrus and strawberry flavours. Many other synthetics were created along with perfumes over the decades, turning the company into a titan in the field, its reputation cemented by one of its in-house chemists winning the Nobel Prize in chemistry in 1939.

Leopold Ružička had been the company's Director of Research and Development when his work on polymethylenes, some of the most common plastic substances still used in packing today, and his work elucidating the structures of many hormones, including the creation of the very first synthetic androgen (a male sex hormone) catapulted the company into fragrance superstardom with an annual turnover today of nearly 4 billion Swiss francs.

Today, neuroscience, physiology and psychology researchers are aided by sensory analysis via artificial intelligence and machine learning and they have made some game-changing discoveries in their field. One, in a circuitous way, helped demystify my nose's strange response to the little bottle of jasmine.

The answer lay with indole, an aromatic compound found in the fragrance produced by the jasmine flower. Chemists will explain at length that indole is a heterocyclic compound built with a six-piece benzene ring fused to a five-membered nitrogen-containing pyrrole ring. If this means nothing, suffice to say that in its isolated form indole stinks – pretty much like poo, although some people describe it as a musty, wet stink while others can even perceive it as sharp, penetrating and also strangely clean. Mason Hainey, a small bespoke perfumer in the US, wrote memorably of indole as an 'odd combination, wet dog, stale hot breath and mothballs all rolled into one'.

Once upon a time, perfume houses captured the smell of jasmine through the ancient process of enfleurage, in which flowers were hand-picked and pressed into layers of fat to allow the scent to migrate from the dying petals into the oily layer from where it would be extracted. An estimated 8,000 handpicked flowers are needed to produce a millilitre of oil, making jasmine 'absolut' one of the most expensive ingredients in the world and a luxury only a handful of perfume houses can afford. Indole occurs naturally and is found in all the white florals, including gardenia, tuberose, neroli and orange blossom, but these days it is also man-made and when added in trace amounts loses the horror stench to add what perfumers describe as a seductive or animalic edge to a scent, a biological whiff that appears to attract rather than repulse.

Could it be that as my olfactory epithelium regenerated and the receptors returned to life, that they were responding only to indole and missing the rest of the perfume?

'Jasmine is a chemically and perceptually complex mixture of hundreds of molecules and its chemical constituents are odorants,' Dr Margot said. 'But it is our brain that builds a representation of this mixture.' To illustrate his point, the scientist flicked his PowerPoint presentation to a graphic depicting the chemical make-up of fourteen of the main organic molecules contained in the little white flower's heavenly scent. Each one smells different: one is green and grassy; another leathery; several are floral or fruity notes; others fruity/lactonic or milky; others spicy/clove and balsamic. Indole is described as faecal/animalic.

Dr Margot then dipped a clutch of perfumers' blotters into the indole and passed it around the lecture room: we all took turns smelling it and while the majority described it as stinky faecal, I could smell only the sharp whiff of naphthalene, the key ingredient in mothballs, which reminded me of my grandmother's winter wardrobe. Dr Margot asked us to hang on to the indole blotter while he dipped another batch into something he called Lilyflore and which to all of us smelled gently pleasant and floral. Then he asked us to hold one blotter in each hand, indole left, Lilyflore right, and to bring one then the other slowly towards our noses: at one point, as the two met, the indole/faeces/mothballs disappeared from my nose completely only to be replaced by the gentle floral. In jasmine, indole keeps its individual scent signature. However, under different circumstances, for example if placed together with other fragrant ingredients, indole can lose its smell 'identity' completely thanks to the momentary inhibition of its olfactory receptors.

This, Dr Margot told us, is an example of the use of a synthetic aromatic compound that has been built to act as an antagonist in our receptors to another: what he called Lilyflore is a compound patented in 2017 by Firmenich literally to block the malodour of the indole. And this, in simple form, is the basis for a particularly significant discovery, one that has humanitarian not just aesthetic implications and which is already helping to improve the health of millions of people in developing or war-torn nations. I remember reading about it when billionaire philanthropist Bill Gates spoke about the sanitation challenges faced by the world: one billion people have no access to toilets and defecate in the open, 3 billion more have toilets but their waste is dumped untreated, seeping into water supplies and leading to the death of 800,000 children each year, felled by cholera and unsafe waters.

As a reporter, I have visited refugee camps where thousands of people are packed into close quarters and the smell of mass latrines is akin to being kicked in the gut by a horse. It is a terrible, inescapable mix of the bitter ammonia of rancid urine, sweat and faeces, often intensified by heat. It is understandable that people in such situations try to find a private space and some dignity wherever else they can. Toilet smells are complicated, often containing more than 200 different compounds and they change over time and depending on temperatures and diets. Dr Margot and his team wanted first to isolate the worst culprits and this is where indole, butyric acid (that parmesan smell) and a couple of others reared their ugly heads. They then tried to recreate the stench, what Gates cheerfully described as 'poop perfume', to test it with people at home in Switzerland and then in India and Africa to see which one best mimicked a stinking toilet. With the poo parfum in hand, they then threw themselves into finding a way to block the smell: as a fragrance company with 125 years of work under its belt battling everything from wet dogs and rugs to smelly armpits, it was best placed to try. But the aim was not to sweep the smell under the carpet and mask it; they wanted to develop a compound that blocked rather than excited its specific olfactory receptors, a similar process to noise-cancelling headphones. The two little blotters in front of our noses showed us the result of olfactory molecular science in action.

Dr Margot is a chemist by training but he describes his professional raison d'être as trying to unravel the links between emotion and smell. He wants to understand why a candle infused with a citrus smell can be enlivening, as if the air had been refreshed and cleansed, while a cinnamon candle evokes cosy comfort, a sense of being in front of the fireplace, hot chocolate in hand.

A large part of his work revolves around testing, examining and explaining human responses to smells including some pioneering work with MRIs that showed that while we might consciously perceive the jasmine odour as pleasant holistically, different parts of our brain light up showing that the neurological process requires identification of both the pleasant and unpleasant separately.[1] The company is building an ever-growing database of research on culture-specific smell response and memories. During Covid and the earliest wave of global lockdowns, it launched a vast survey across eleven nations revealing that the very same fragrance can have a completely different effect on consumers depending on which part of the world they come from.

If you want to test these findings yourself, think about what 'clean' smells like for you. In my mind, it is the pungent odour of bleach or ammonia because it reminds me of my grandmother's house in Italy, when windows were thrown open to the sunshine, carpets aired and clean sheets dried on the line. In London, it's rare to encounter this cleaning product alone as it is perceived to be a little too brutal but occasionally, holidaying in southern Italy or Greece, you smell it in the early morning as you walk past freshly washed, whitewashed doorsteps or in the local taverna loo. I am immediately transported to the sensation of being somewhere glistening with cleanliness.

If you ask an American the same question, the chances are they will mention the smell of pine. Despite the fact that pine sap is sticky and stains and makes a big mess, North American consumers have used a cleaning product called Pine Sol since the late 1920s, mopping their floors and scrubbing kitchens and it remains a favourite with Americans surveyed about smells they feel have 'germ-killing, deep-cleaning' powers. In Southeast Asia, from Indonesia to Thailand and Vietnam, it is different again: it's the scent of lemon, lime and lemongrass that evokes cleanliness and the elimination of bacteria. I know first hand that not far away in Australia, where I lived for many years, consumers gravitate towards eucalyptus and tea-tree scents gathered from the huge, evergreen trees that are abundant and indigenous to the great island continent.

Firmenich wanted to analyse responses to try to decode what scents made consumers feel safe and clean at a time when the world was gripped by fear and uncertainty about disease and infection and the dramatic changes in social interaction and lifestyle. While much of it remains top secret and is patented for their clients, it revealed that particularly at a time of insecurity, familiar scents and smells that evoke good memories offer solace. Of the 6,400 people surveyed, some 56 per cent of respondents from eleven countries reported that not only did they appreciate the impact of smell more since lockdown but that they took more comfort from scents and fragrances. Almost 70 per cent admitted that quarantine at home had had a big impact on their well-being, reporting a range of emotions, from fear, anger and insecurity to the positive desire to nest, care and love those around them more.

Ilaria Resta, the company's Perfumery Global President said fragrances have long reinforced feelings of happiness and calm but this was magnified for consumers facing stressful situations, prompting the company to document the smells that evoke safety and cleanliness, and naming this rollcall of molecular combinations of scents Sereni-Clean. She predicted these may well remain in consumers' minds for some time – and I suspect she might well be right.

23

Smelly Stories of Art and Industry

Movie producers have also long been fascinated by the potential for using smell to enhance the cinematic experience, although the very first attempts to harness olfaction were not to entice and delight audiences but to keep disgusted viewers in their seats.

Poor ventilation and low ceilings in the first purpose-built cinemas of the early twentieth century meant that the malodour of several hundred bodies crammed in together quickly became a distraction. At first, 'air breaks', a kind of breather interval, were introduced; theatres added fragrant fountains in their lobbies, and staff deodorised with a mothball scent called Perolin during screenings. One cinema in Berlin even used an electronically driven balloon to spray a fragrance over the heads of their smelly customers. More than a century later the German multinational Bosch produced 'FreshUp', an electronic device no bigger than an old-fashioned clothes brush, which uses plasma molecules to remove, rather than simply mask, stale smells such as smoke and body odour from fabrics.

The first 'atmospheric' use of scent during film was in 1906 during a Newsreel screening of the Pasadena Rose Parade in Pennsylvania when the essence of roses was blown through fans into a theatre, using cotton balls dipped in a scented liquid. There are no reports about how it was received by the public although four years earlier, a German-Japanese poet named Sadakichi Hartmann staged the world's first scent performance in New York. It was titled *A Trip to Japan in Sixteen Minutes* and he was booed off the stage, the audience apparently put off by his waving of fragrance-soaked fabrics in front of a fan, accompanied by two kimono-clad women.

Over the next three decades there would be sporadic interest in technology that aimed to synchronise 'narrative' scents, including cutting notches into film to trigger the timed release of various appropriate fragrances ,while a Swiss company produced 'odorated talking pictures' and the film *My Dream* for the 1940 New York World's Fair promised the timed spraying of twenty odours using an air-cooling system. Walt Disney was also tempted to the olfactory, originally envisioning his 1940 animated feature *Fantasia* as a sensory filmgoing experience, not just of sight and sound but using scent effects. In the end, the cost and onerous logistics stopped him going ahead.

In the early 1960s, the LSD generation re-aroused interest in smell and performance, welcoming the arrival of sensory technologies including AromaRama, Smell-O-Vision, Odorama scratch-and-sniff cards and Scent-A-Vision, which would later be used with so-called '4D tech', which included motion seats, wind and fog machines. None of them lasted long, regarded by audiences and critics as gimmickry or marketing stunts rather than as a true sensory enrichment of the visual experience. In the end, faulty technology added to the failures as machines worked intermittently, wafting a citrus smell across the cinema as, onscreen, an orange was sliced open but too often descending into olfactory chaos when glitches such as the smell of freshly mown grass lingered over a vista of the sands of the Gobi Desert.

In the early 1960s, what could best be described as an early video game, brainchild of experimental filmmaker Morton Heilig, would be seen as the birth of virtual-reality genres and hailed for its great potential. A patent drawing of Heilig's 'Sensorama' simulator shows the viewer seated with his or her head inside a box-like viewing screen. The game offered players the 3D-film experience of riding a motorbike through the streets of Brooklyn, the wind blowing through their hair, vibrations of the seat beneath them, and all this accompanied by the changing smells of a big metropolis. Heilig's vision didn't make it to production: once again, the costs of this kind of sensory filmmaking were too high and his vision too imaginative and complex for the marketers. Heilig had foreseen a future for the cinema that would see 'the air filled with odours. We will feel changes in temperature and the texture of things. We will feel physically transported into a new world.' But it would take another seventy years for his ideas to come to fruition.

✦

London filmmaker Grace Boyle runs a company creating multi-sensory content that she says brings perfumery, perception science, creative technologists and artistic installation in the world of XR together. She calls the project 'The Feelies', a reference to Aldous Huxley's futuristic musical instrument, the scent organ.

In his seminal 1932 novel *Brave New World* the strange contraption played

> a delightfully refreshing Herbal Capriccio – rippling arpeggios of thyme and lavender, of rosemary, basil, myrtle, tarragon; a series of daring modulations through the spice keys into ambergris; and a slow return through sandalwood, camphor, cedar and newly mown hay (with the occasional subtle touches of discord – a whiff of kidney pudding, the faintest suspicion of pig's dung) back to the simple aromatics with which the piece began.

One of Boyle's major works has been the award-winning virtual-reality film *Munduruku: The fight to defend the heart of the Amazon*, a campaign video produced for Greenpeace, which follows the struggle of the indigenous Munduruku people, whose lands in the Tapajos river basin are threatened by large-scale industrial projects including a hydroelectric dam that would flood the rainforest. Instead of odour being added as an afterthought, relegating it to a gimmick, the concept was 'baked' into the script, even taking a perfumer on set to map the smells of a rainforest. The result was a virtual-reality film in which the viewer sits in a high-tech version of Heilig's Sensorama as they are transported into the heart of village life in all its earthy, organic heat and the complex array of scents that define the great forest and its ecosystems. The story then shifts to depict the threat and stench of industrialisation defined by choking machine and diesel fumes, burned rubber tyres and even the acrid sweat of the workforce. Boyle's company also worked on an immersive installation at the Saatchi Gallery in

London titled *We live in an ocean of air*, which asked viewers to wear VR masks and explore the trunk of a giant sequoia tree, experiencing it from inside and out, starting with the earthy smell of its root system upward through the trunk and into its branches and leaves. Breath became visible as it bubbled and turned red to represent the exchange of oxygen and carbon dioxide. 'We need to design experiences with every sense – visual should not be elevated above any other. Scent can immediately transport us in place and time, and that power cannot be ignored,' she said.

The Austrian artist, inventor and environmental activist Wolfgang Georgsdorf says he began his foray into olfactory art '170 years after moving pictures began' while he was still a student at art school in Linz. A solid man with a tanned, bald head and a penchant for wearing funky-coloured braces, Georgsdorf hums with an unrequited energy and seems to flash rather than walk across a room like some kind of manic forest spirit.

'I once conducted an orchestra playing [an arrangement of] Schubert's *Trout Quintet* and cooked some fish in the performances and threw trout into the audience. Smell is a link and bridge between many things,' he tells me. Georgsdorf thinks his fascination with the effect of smell on the imagination and memory began when he was about four years old. Many in his family were medics and biologists, his grandfather an analyst chemist, and he remembers begging to be allowed to hang onto a pile of out-of-date medication that was destined for the garbage:

> When I asked if I could keep it, they told me I could die
> if I ate the stuff . . . I told them I didn't want to eat it, I
> just wanted to smell it all! They gave me flasks and cough

drops and all sorts of things and I moved them around and changed their order and smelled and smelled them and there was my first olfactory pan flute.

That's a true story and smell has always intrigued me, how it is perceived, what people think is beautiful or terrible or strong and at what threshold. I played music, I drew and painted, I made sculptures and built things but, somehow, I've been working with smells for years: it connected all these disciplines for me.

Georgsdorf has spent more than three decades building and perfecting several prototypes of what he calls the 'Smeller', a machine that in its first incarnation could best be described as a scent organ with mechanical levers that pumped out smells. His Smeller 2.0 has evolved into a sophisticated, multi-channel electronically controlled instrument or sculptural machine with which he composes and tells stories via scent. Fragrant symphonies? Smelly stories? No, odour drama. In 2016, he founded Osmodrama – from the ancient Greek 'osmo' for smell and 'drama' which meant plot – or 'Storytelling with Scents', the first festival of kinetic scent performance in Europe in St Johannes Evangelist Church in the centre of Berlin. The programme spanned art forms and included literary readings, musical performance, films synchronised to scent and workshops bringing together olfactory scientists with artists to talk about smell.

The most recent Smeller 2.0 looks like a cross between an enormous daisy and a cluster of cannons and while Georgsdorf deliberately tried to build it around utilitarian requirements so the visual experience did not overtake the olfactory, in photographs at least I find it very, very beautiful. He describes it simply as a 'functional artwork' containing sixty-four channels. It can be 'played' in the way a DJ would plan a set but rather than plugging in a speaker, Georgsdorf plugs in the Smeller.

The vision and drive to bring smell to art has never been easy: the machines are costly to build, difficult to install, require large, well-ventilated gallery or museum spaces and funding. Artistic patronage is always hard to secure. 'We need spaces that are not too big but also not too small that allow us to have control over the air, whirl-proof spaces. It started as a scientific project with an artistic drive because there weren't any prerequisite technical gadgets to help perform it and we often failed,' he told me.

'Now, we are building a cocoon of white parachute silk in a church in Berlin to experiment with time-based performances that can be co-related to cinema, to dance and literature.' Over the years, Georgsdorf's perseverance and sheer force of will has seen him exhibit, perform and collaborate with an array of Europe's most interesting contemporary artists and in important museums and art galleries, including the Gropius Bau in Berlin. However, he is particularly proud of forging a theoretical discussion between art and science, working with deaf communities and often performing with no text and no images, just the sensory input of the Osmodrama via Smeller 2.0.

Osmodrama also brought Georgsdorf to Professor Thomas Hummel's attention; he has lectured at the International Centre for Smell and Taste at Dresden Hospital for several years, also testing theories that exposure to smells and odour-driven storytelling might have a positive impact on those suffering both anosmia and depression. I participated in a kind of test performance in which he and his young protégé and budding perfumer-assistant, Kasper Helml, used a fan and enacted the passage of time with a battery of natural animal and earthy smells that gradually succumbed to the stench of industrialisation, smoke-belching factories and old batteries. Wearing earplugs and noise-cancelling headphones along with black goggles, it was an extraordinary experience – both bewildering and enlightening as my brain seemed to need to shift gears to perceive the world through this single sense. Georgsdorf explained the thinking behind the performance:

> Smells work because they help to revitalise people's emotional life at both a conscious and subconscious level. We hold onto pictures, experiences in memory and smells evoke responses in the oldest part of the brain, the one where there is no reason or judgement involved, just feeling.
>
> In art, this attempt to compose and to perform and to tell stories with thousands of scents and smells has not existed. I am obsessed, I am fascinated by the idea that I can paint pictures not for the eyes but behind the eyes with invisible things and where the imagination makes the object as it does reading literature or hearing music.

❋

Where artists such as Georgsdorf dream of using smell to awaken the human imagination, ignite emotions and aesthetic pleasure for the sheer sake of experience, the world of commerce is increasingly focused on finding out how best to use smell to sell. Close your eyes and picture a group of children playing basketball. Can you hear the pitched squeak as they pivot and turn, their sneakers skidding on the polished timber court? Can you smell the mix of oil and rubber? That's what Nike wants its customers to sniff as they shop for a new set of trainers. Or how about the crisp scent of a freshly ironed cotton shirt or the smell of Christmas – but not pine needles and mulled wine; rather, the winter comforts of sitting by a fire in an old leather chair with a glass of cognac. These are just a few of the synthetic molecular aromas being created to market products through our noses.

This very specific niche of commercial research was officially named aromachology in the late 1980s when the Fragrance Foundation, the non-profit, educational arm of the international perfume industry, set up a group of scientists to study the influence of odours on human behaviour and to examine the relationship between smell and emotion. Over the last three decades the commercial application of olfaction has become big business. It's not enough any more to spray any old perfume into the air or channel the smell of bread-baking through shops and hotels via an air-conditioning system; the scents have to be subtle and targeted, even changed from season to season as a department store changes its stock, or hour to hour according to the shopping habits of customers. One US department store reported that sales went up when vanilla was sprayed through the women's clothing department and a rose fragrance through menswear, but when the scents were reversed sales plummeted, prompting ongoing investigation into why.

One of the Fragrance Foundation's most recent studies concluded that 65 per cent of consumers can recall what they smelled in a store after a year. This compares to barely 50 per cent who can recall what they saw just three months before. The results echo a study by Rockefeller University that found that people can recall 35 per cent of what they smell compared to 5 per cent of what they see, 2 per cent of what they hear and 1 per cent of what they touch.

Hotel chains often use scent combinations pumped through lobbies to imprint their brand on guests. The Westin chain, for example, uses a blend of white tea, wood cedar and vanilla to represent a 'cool and relaxing' atmosphere. The St Regis prefers rose, sweet pea and pipe tobacco to define 'elegance' and the W Hotels group entices a younger clientele with lime and lemon blossom. Edition Hotel in Times Square in New York wanted to play to its arty, eclectic interiors and chose black tea, citrus, smoke, chocolate and pepper.

Scent branding is a key ingredient of retail marketing strategy, encouraged by dozens of surveys, studies and focus groups that continue to analyse shopper behaviour and hone the use of artificial scents to influence the time customers spend browsing, the purchases they make, even how much they are prepared to spend.

The famed French shopping mall Galeries Lafayette experimented with fragrance and questioned shoppers about their perceptions. Without a scent in the air, those surveyed guessed accurately that they had spent thirty minutes in store, but once a fragrance was introduced, shoppers spent more than an hour browsing but believed they had been inside just twenty-five minutes. Luxury-car manufacturers enhance the perception of decadence by spraying 'essence of leather' through their new vehicles; music company Sony uses an 'olfactory logo' of mandarin orange to define an elegance, combined with bourbon and vanilla to appeal to men and women respectively.

The men's clothing company Abercrombie & Fitch set out to find a scent that defined 'rugged individualism' for its stores – although Covid has since moved them online. Valentino uses a scent signature titled 'Effortless Grace' mixing rose, citrus, jasmine and leather while Hugo Boss opted for a minimalist, woody fragrance.

Mindful of humans' sharp sense of smell but low recall when faced with more than three odours, some companies have deliberately settled on a single aroma to define their place in the market. The athletic shoe shop chain Footlocker settled on grapefruit, a smell it felt matched its youthful image, while Harrods in rainy London uses beachy coconut oil smells in its women's swimwear department and the fruit of ancient legends, pomegranate, in the luxury accessories section. If you ever feel hungry in John Lewis's kitchen appliance section, it is probably because the retailer releases the smell of a warm, sweet nougat to stimulate the appetite while you're browsing. The sales tricks are endless.

When confectioner Hershey's opened in Times Square in New York they experimented by spraying a chocolate fragrance through the store. Marketers were delighted when sales rose 34 per cent, encouraging them to attach scented strips to their vending machines. The Hard Rock Cafe chain uses the artificial smell of cookies and waffle cones, while Disney World gets the saliva going with a 'grill scent' to make its frozen burgers appear freshly flipped from a wood barbecue. Head & Shoulders shampoo returned to the old scratch-and-sniff card in a print advertisement campaign to entice consumers to test its 'apple fresh' fragrances, while frozen-food giant McCain installed tech to spread the smell of baking potatoes at selected bus stops across the UK, hoping to entice customers to buy its range of jacket potatoes.

The rush for olfactory branding is now a billion-dollar industry. Apart from multinational titans such as Givaudan and Firmenich, it has also spawned niche scent specialists including twin sisters Dawn and Samantha Goldworm, who started their New York company 12.29 after 'scenting a handbag' for the luxury Italian fashion house, Bottega Veneta. The sisters now count companies including Nike, American Express and Cadillac among their clients, as well as stars such as singer Lady Gaga.

It was Dawn who created the Nike scent and the complex 'crisp fresh' fragrance for shirt manufacturer Pye, which combined orris (made from the root of iris flowers), woody papyrus, pink pepper, smooth sandalwood and musk: 'It's all about an emotional response,' she says. 'We dissect all of the brand cues – the aesthetics, the sound, the shapes and the target market – and translate that into a smell that responds on a generational, cultural and environmental basis.'

British Airways has long used a mix of scents evoking freshly cut grass and sea air in its airport lounges and then also in aircraft. But there is an additional challenge for airlines. At altitude, food tastes are largely dulled in the artificial environment created by a combination of pressurised cabins, dry air and background noise that dulls the sense of smell and, as a result, perception of flavour. Studies have also shown that there is even an effect on the tongue and how travellers perceive the five tastes at altitude.

The use of scent has also found its way into workplaces where, rather than lull shoppers into spending more time and money in a fragrant haze, management would like to stimulate the workforce into greater productivity. The Japanese construction company Takasago Corporation found that spraying lavender through its offices reduced keyboard errors by 20 per cent, although jasmine (33 per cent) and lemon (54 per cent) were even more effective.[1]

Rather than aiming at increased productivity, a women-only working space in New York called The Wing has used scent – a combination of milk, steamed rice, iris and sandalwood – to evoke a sense of comfort and safety.

Olivia Jezler, a perfumer who used to create scents for fragrance and fashion houses including Christian Dior, Victoria's Secret and corporates such as the World Economic Forum, now runs a programme called Scentsplorations, which uses scent to reduce anxiety, enhance alertness and elevate mood. She conceived the idea of a workshop because of the impact of Covid and now runs group sessions during which participants, usually from the same workplace, embark on a series of 'cross-sensory exercises' using everyday objects such as books and even fresh laundry, designed to stimulate conversation.

'It's a tonic for Covid, I suppose,' she says from her home in New York.

> People have struggled to find the motivation to work, especially through this strange period, which has raised anxiety levels. I caught Covid myself and had a brief period where I lost my sense of smell. I noticed it because I couldn't smell peppermints on my desk and went through a few days of weirdness before it started to come back.

People aren't conscious of what they are smelling or why they like it. In the workshop they talk about memories, so people end up sharing stories and connecting. And because our language for smells is so limited it means they have to move away from business jargon and find other ways of expressing those feelings. It gets people out of their own space, working with others and builds things like innovation.

24

Tip of the Iceberg

In 1914, Alexander Graham Bell, the inventor of the telephone, made a speech to the graduating class of the Friends' School in Washington on the theme of 'discovery and invention'. In his address, published a month later in *National Geographic* magazine, he challenged his audience with a surprising question:

> What is an odour? Is it an emanation of material particles into the air, or is it a form of vibration, like sound? Did you ever try to measure a smell? Can you tell whether one smell is just as strong as another? It is very obvious that we have many different kinds of smells, all the way from the odour of violets and roses up to asafoetida (the gum of a type of fennel which smells like rotten garlic). But until you measure their likeness and differences you can have no science of odour . . . and if you are ambitious to found a new science, then measure a smell.[1]

I read Bell's prescient, promise-filled words not long after returning from my week-long immersion in the world of

251

twenty-first-century olfactory research in Dresden. Were he alive now, what would the inventor make of our century's countless, ground-breaking discoveries about the mysterious fifth sense? Would he be fascinated and elated by the unfathomable complexity and richness unearthed by this new olfactory science or would he be bewildered by just how much we still don't know?

Extraordinary as it may sound, one of the most important of these finds emerged into the public spotlight while I was in Germany when a team of researchers at Rockefeller University in New York published a revolutionary paper that provides the very first view – at molecular level – of exactly how an odour molecule binds to an olfactory receptor.[2]

For many biologists working in the olfactory field, seeing this process with their own eyes is akin to the Holy Grail, taking them a step closer to understanding how the hell it is that animals and humans can discriminate between such an inordinate number of smells.

But nobody had yet clapped eyes on what actually happens at the level of the molecule itself until the Rockefeller team decided to place one of the most evolutionarily primitive insects on earth, the jumping bristletail, in the sights of one of the world's most advanced and revolutionary imaging techniques. Known as cryo-electron microscopy, the process requires the freezing of biomolecules in living cells while they're in mid-motion, which in turn allows resolution of 3D images at the level of the atom. Its development won three scientists (Cambridge's Richard Henderson, Columbia's Joachim Frank and the University of Lausanne's Jacques Dubochet) a shared Nobel Prize in 2017. For the record, jumping bristletails are ground-dwelling bugs believed to have appeared in the Middle Devonian period, around the same time as spiders, and look a little like common silverfish or tiny, air-breathing prawns.

Scientists have long studied insect olfactory systems as they are relatively simple and rely on specialised proteins acting as a passageway (known as an ion channel) for electrical signals. To date, more than one million insect species have been identified on Earth and each one has developed a different set of proteins and a passageway specific to its environment and needs. Like animals, insects must process an array of general smells and identify the ones important for survival.

Led by the brilliant young neuroscientist Professor Vanessa Ruta, the Rockefeller team decided to try to capture the behaviour of the jumping bristletails' receptors as they were exposed to different odorants in a bid to begin to explain how a finite number of receptors can detect 'an almost infinite chemical world'. The first odorant used was common eugenol (which humans perceive as a clove-like smell) and the second was a compound used as an insect repellent and which is known as diethyltoluamide (DEET). The molecules of each are very different structurally and yet the researchers quickly realised that both docked onto the very same pocket in the binding receptor. What they didn't expect was that the substance lining the pockets didn't form strong chemical bonds with the smell and rather than appearing to be good chemical matches, they were more like 'friendly acquaintances'.

Ruta observed that these kinds of non-specific chemical interactions offered the freedom for many more different odorants to be recognised. In other words, rather than responding to a single chemical feature, they were more flexible and responded in a holistic way, recognising the general chemical nature of the smell. Ruta's team was able to see that the receptor seemed to recognise each molecule for itself, rather than each one being a perfect chemical match. When the researchers widened the receptor pocket, it showed a stronger response to DEET, which is a larger molecule itself but it also lessened its affinity to the clove smell, which perhaps was not able to snuggle into a bigger pocket quite as closely.

The receptor's 'promiscuity', Ruta observed, doesn't rule out its ability to be highly specific either. 'Although each receptor responds to a large number of molecules, it's insensitive to others,' she said. Equally interesting was the observation that when they tweaked the amino acids in the pocket, this changed the receptor as well as the molecules with which it prefers to bind. Ruta and her team believe that this flexibility helps to explain how insects have been able to evolve, adapting quickly to their specific environments.

Harvard's Professor Bob Datta describes the work as pioneering and an 'unequivocally landmark paper', although Professor Ruta, who described what she saw as rather 'beautiful', insists there is still much to learn: 'It is the first structure of odorant recognition in any receptor from any species. But it's probably not the only mechanism of odorant recognition . . . it's just one solution to the problem – and very unlikely that it's the only solution.'

※

As I thought more about this discovery and Alexander Graham Bell's entreaty to the students about establishing a science of smell, it dawned on me that he too had lived through a terrible pandemic. Spanish influenza exploded across the globe just four years after his speech, killing an estimated 50 million people and wreaking the effects of this mysterious illness on a third of the world's population.

In 1996, the remains of seven coal miners lost to Spanish flu in 1918 were found buried in permafrost in Spitsbergen, a Norwegian island in the Arctic Circle, and identified from records. They were exhumed by researchers from the US and Canada, allowing the removal and examination of frozen lung tissue to identify the pathogen likely to have caused the pandemic. Genomic testing would reveal that this particular virus probably originated in birds and was an ancestor of classical swine and human H1N1 influenzas.[3] Anosmia was not reported during the Spanish influenza pandemic although thousands of survivors were later struck by a concurrent neurological condition, 'encephalitis lethargica', more commonly known at the time as the sleeping sickness. Clinicians now believe that this strain of the influenza virus also attacked the central nervous system through the nose and led to a three-fold increase in incidents of Parkinson's disease among people born between 1881 and 1924.[4]

Today, the loss of smell is much more widely well known to be a signal that the nervous system has been implicated in an infection. It acts as a red flag to physicians looking out for the earliest, non-motor symptoms of Parkinson's disease – and of course, it is formally accepted as a primary symptom of Covid-19.

And yet according to Professor Marc Van Ranst, a Belgian coronavirus expert, the world has experienced an epidemic of smell loss before – and not so long ago either. Van Ranst and fellow Belgian and German researchers suspect that the Russian flu epidemic that spread from St Petersburg into Europe and to the United States in the 1890s felling thousands was not caused by an influenza virus at all.

§

In my quest to find out more about the internal structures of our olfactory system, I spent a fascinating morning in Dresden examining a human brain with Rostock University's Anatomy Professor, Martin Witt. After showing us how to identify sections of the olfactory bulb and epithelium of newborn mice and a frontal section of human glomeruli under the microscope, we gathered around a stainless steel workbench. Over the next hour, Witt seemed to take secret delight in watching our faces as he removed a brain from a bucket filled with preservation liquids and offered us the opportunity to hold it in our hands. After a deep breath, I was surprised by its weight and resilience to the touch as well as awestruck by the opportunity to observe in real life what we normally only see in a textbook. Not long after, I had to breathe even more deeply when he lifted a human head from its container, revealing it had been halved vertically to reveal the olfactory system in all its mind-boggling complexity. When he laid it gently onto a stainless-steel tray, the ear and empty eye socket were revealed, providing visual signposts to its humanity and giving me a brief, existential shock. However, sheer fascination quickly took over as Professor Witt used his scalpel to point out and encourage us to identify the key structures essential for smell: the olfactory bulbs, piriform cortex, amygdala and hippocampus.

The process took me back to the words of Professor Basile Landis, Director of Head and Neck Surgery at University

Hospitals of Geneva, who reminded us that we should always think of the nose as 'the tip of the iceberg'. 'What you see is just the external architecture . . . what's really interesting is what lies underneath,' he said. As I focused on the stark reality of the cadaver in front of me, I remembered too that he had likened the nose to a 'corridor with many doors of varying sizes leading to smaller rooms containing very different furniture'. Sure enough, I could look into the skull and follow the trajectory of convoluted, pink, slightly stringy labyrinthine channels in this way. The sinuses are encountered first even if 'science still has no real answer for what they're good for', Landis had observed. The septum, the structure that divides the long space comes next while the turbinates, small ante-rooms, sit off the sides of the 'corridor'. I could identify these slightly odd protuberances too, knowing they were designed by nature to add surface area to the nose because unlike a toilet pipe that needs to be straight and clear to work, the nose needs to slow down incoming air so it can clean, humidify and settle it to body temperature before it enters the lungs.

'It's 23 degrees today and humidity is about 40 per cent,' Landis had told us. 'The nose will transform that air to ensure it is 30 degrees and 100 per cent humidity in seconds. Try to breathe for an hour just through your mouth to test this process: you will feel dry, full of dust, incredibly uncomfortable.'

Now, as I looked at the dissected head lying on Professor Witt's tray, it took on the qualities of a 3D cutaway, colour graphic, allowing me to share Professor Landis's sense of wonder. Here, in this tiny space, wrapped securely in bone and cartilage for protection, is an astonishing organ, an entire system capable of performing an inordinate and varied number of physiological functions. It allows us to breathe, to smell and perceive myriad odours and flavour, alerts us to imminent danger, and has specialist nerves to protect and get rid of unwanted foreign substances. The nose produces special hormones as shields, known as cilia cells that can move and kill bacteria, erectile blood vessels capable of swelling like sexual organs to respond to irritants and regulate air flow. And it helps give our voices resonance, offers a sophisticated air-conditioning service and cycles every sixty minutes, so that one side keeps on working while the other rests – not that we know why, but it probably explains the side you choose to sleep.

'My take-home message is simple: the nose is not a homogenous organ. Every breath you take, the body and brain checks all of this passively, without consulting you,' concluded Professor Landis with just the slightest hint of a grin. 'God formed man from the dust of the ground and breathed into his nostrils to make him a living being . . . even the Bible puts the nose at the centre of Creation.'

25

Hope in the Time
of Anosmia

One of the toughest aspects of anosmia in the wake of injury, viral infection and now Covid as well is that no doctor on earth can possibly tell you how long it will last or, indeed, if you will recover at all. As I write this, over 500 million people around the world have been infected with Covid and at least half will have experienced a smell or taste disturbance. Ten per cent of those, like me, will suffer persistent symptoms and we still don't know how many will never recover their fifth sense. When I was infected, so early in the pandemic, I'd instinctively had to adopt Benjamin Disraeli's philosophy of being 'prepared for the worst but hope for the best' because so very little was known about the novel virus let alone how the olfactory system would respond. Less than eighteen months later, not only do we have a suite of vaccines – and that is the other great science story of the twenty-first century – but thanks to Bob Datta's lab at Harvard, we know how the virus gets in and his colleagues around the world are helping us to come ever closer to understanding exactly how it turns off our sense of smell. Datta told me:

This is the truly emerging science but already there are some exciting hypotheses. Stavros Lomvardas [Professor of Biochemistry and Molecular Biophysics at Columbia] did the same kind of experiment I did, but on actual human tissue. And he too confirms there is no evidence that the virus infects the sensory neurones and that it is the support cells that are hit.

But they can go even further and see that the sensory neurones seem to sense local inflammation and respond, for example, by changing the expression of genes needed to sense odour . . . in other words they turn down the genes responsible for smell. So there is a lot more science still to be done but this has the feel of a likely hypothesis.

Apart from the groups of drugs used to treat the most common nasal disorders (steroids, antihistamines, decongestants) there is nothing to treat loss of smell itself. Despite this, anecdotal evidence from the avalanche of desperate patients posting daily on social media anosmia-support groups showed that in Europe but particularly in the United States, many ENT doctors and GPs had resorted to prescribing corticosteroid sprays to their patients. This may be understandable as medics want to address their patients' anxieties and symptoms but these were clinical decisions taken on the hoof with no scientific backing. Disturbed by the lack of evidence-based treatment options, an international group of clinical olfactory specialists, including the University of East Anglia's Professor Carl Philpott and others we have met – Thomas Hummel, Alexander Fjældstad, Basile Landis – decided to take matters into their own hands. Over a period of months, they embarked on a forensic, collaborative and international review of all the existing, published and peer-reviewed literature on the treatment of smell disturbances triggered by viruses and then took the unusual step of writing a consensus paper on how best to treat the epidemic of post-Covid anosmics.

Their verdict? After trawling through 467 scientific papers, this eminent group advised against any kind of drug, recommending instead twice-daily smell training – and a good dose of patience.

You will remember that Professor Hummel was the first to experiment with olfactory training with patients three decades ago, asking them to undergo a twice-daily regime in which they sniffed four different smells: rose, clove, lemon and eucalyptus. At the time, his approach had aroused great scepticism among his peers but his early results were encouraging and he and many other clinicians throughout the world have persevered with the 'use it to get it back' approach. In 2009, he conducted a formal twelve-week study with a large group of anosmic patients that showed significant improvement among those that committed to smell training and since then there have been several other trials that have all documented statistically significant enhancements in patients' smell identification and thresholds. While none of these experiments has been of the gold-standard, randomised-controlled type of trial, smell training is a treatment that doesn't require prescription, can be done at home easily and cheaply and, most importantly, carries no dangers of side-effects or harm.

In the UK, both charities – AbScent and Fifth Sense – offer guidance on how to smell train. You can use essential-oil kits bought ready made, make your own or even use simple ingredients you might have at home. AbScent's Chrissi Kelly says the ideal home-made kit requires four little screw-top dark-glass jars, some artist's watercolour blotting paper and the four oils you choose to smell. Cut a round piece of the paper to fit the bottom of the little jar and add a single drop of the oil:

> A good place to put your jars is beside your bed, then it's a reminder every day as you wake up or before you go to sleep to do your smell training. Each time, open the jar, hold it close but not on your nose. Take a few quick, gentle bunny-style sniffs for 20 seconds, no more. Now, really think and focus on what you are trying to smell. Concentrate as much as you can on really 'finding' that smell. Then relax, take a couple of breaths and move on to the next fragrance until you've done all four.

She tells those she is training that every single time they go through this process, they must try as hard as they can to find a smell signal, persevering even if there is nothing or if it is very weak. Finding an analogy to get through this very discouraging period can also be helpful: for example, imagining that you've thrown a pebble into a well of water but as you've no idea how deep the well might be, you must pay full attention to hear the splash at the bottom. 'You have to try to engage the higher part of your brain to try to remember what that smell might be like . . . as if you were there, at the well, straining to hear the pebble drop. That's how you have to engage with this little jar of smell.'

I know exactly what she means by the need to use every fibre of your being to 'refind' the smell. A large pump bottle of my favourite hand cream, the one that told me I'd become anosmic that horrible March afternoon, still sits beside my bed. I spent more than a year using it as my sentinel as, day in and day out, I placed a pea-size blob onto my hands and sniffed in an effort to retrieve its heady spice and floral scent. Chrissi and many experts suggest that smelling familiar scents is particularly helpful and knowing what you are smelling is imperative. Stimulation of the parts of the brain related to olfaction also appears to be improved if you use more powerful or concentrated odours but be sure to label the jars and ensure the lids don't get mixed up and mingle the scents.

'People who lose their sense of smell often respond by turning away from smell,' Kelly says. 'They stop interrogating their environment, so they go outdoors and don't ask themselves what the day smells like, what flowers and the grass smells like. Smell-training kits help get you back into the habit of smelling again.'

In the end, smell training is a form of recovery based on neuroplasticity, the brain's ability to reorganise itself and compensate for a change or injury. It is widely studied in the rehabilitation of patients who have lost motor or speech functions due, for example, to stroke. Additional recent research with olfaction and smell training suggests that changing the selection of odours every three months can also be useful. And most researchers and clinicians who have studied the results also agree that the longer the training goes on, the better.

I and so many others have had to learn that there is no instant result and smell doesn't get switched back on the way Covid so brutally turned it off. Patience is key.

Reading about the brain's extraordinary ability to make up for injuries in other regions of the body reminded me of a chat with Professor David Laing, the Scottish-born, Australian olfactory researcher, who had told me with a wry smile that neuroscientists working in the chemosensory sphere often say that it is not the nose that smells, nor the ears that hear nor eyes that see: 'It's the brain. The nose, ears and eyes just send electronic signals from their peripheral positions until the brain takes over and does its thing.'

Professor Laing is author of a series of significant experiments commenced in the late 1980s and 1990s which produced seminal evidence that while the human nose can recognise an almost infinite number of individual smells, not even trained 'noses' like perfumers or wine experts can distinguish more than three or four smells once mixed together.[1] I also remembered his appearance on the Australian public broadcaster, the ABC's science programme, *Catalyst*, in which a chef, a wine specialist and a journalist had been invited to see if they could disprove his laboratory's finding. They failed – as has everybody who has tried since. 'We have done a lot of experiments to disprove it ourselves too over the years,' he told me, 'but we have never found anybody that could identify more than four.'

I had not sought Professor Laing out to talk to him about smell training – even though he was also the developer of the world's first smell test designed specifically for children. Rather, I wanted to understand more about a new paper, in which his laboratory offered some hope and a rehabilitation path for patients who have lost their sense of smell after Traumatic Brain Injury (TBI).[2] It was peer reviewed and accepted for publication in June 2021, just as restrictions began to be lifted in the UK and Europe, while Professor Laing was frustratingly locked down at home in Australia before the second stage of his intriguing work could commence.

He explained that the preliminary results rely on the fact that most patients who lose their sense of smell in the wake of a brain injury still have functional gustatory (taste) and trigeminal systems (the latter nerve is the one that responds to chilli or spicy foods, temperature and texture changes). In this group of patients, MRI experiments suggest that it will be possible to bypass the olfactory bulb and activate smell responses/experience directly within the brain. This was first looked at in 2011 by Dr Christina Zelano and colleagues at Northwestern University in Chicago. They were able to show that when subjects with a normal sense of smell were asked to direct their attention to an object with a familiar smell – a lemon, say – the brain generates a predictive search image (in neuroscience speak they call this a neuronal ensemble) in the posterior piriform cortex (PPC).[3] This, they demonstrated, was exactly the same as the 'ensemble' produced when the actual odour was administered, suggesting that by focusing on an odour familiar from memory our brains can produce a version of it merely by retrieving this stored information. In other words, the part of the brain that saves information about smell stimuli and 'reads' them does the same work if the smell is 'real' or imagined. Professor Laing told me:

> The best example on how these search images operate in the brain is if you think about a fox as it is out hunting at night for a rabbit. The fox is sniffing around and cannot see

the rabbit but knows what it smells like; it is familiar with its smell. Familiarity is key in all this. What is happening in the fox's brain is that it is producing search images of the rabbit odour, its brain is pulsing with that information as it is sniffing vigorously and when, suddenly, the real odour enters the nose it reinforces those search images, increasing sensitivity for that odour.

Professor Laing says humans operate in a similar way and his team now wants to show that if a person who has become anosmic due to brain injury is asked to think of an object with a familiar smell – a fish, for instance – a similar process will allow the creation of a 'smell' experience. In humans, the timing is of paramount importance as images are conjured inside three seconds. He explained:

If a person puts a piece of fish in their mouth and starts to chew it, after about three seconds, the odour image will be released and combined with taste signals from the tongue. It is then received by the part of the brain that integrates the two – what you've tasted and smelled – and so the search image of the fish is confirmed. Within seconds, you have an integration of what the fish looks like, tastes like and you are given the information of what it smelled like from the memory centre.

Perhaps, observed Professor Laing, it should not strictly be described as olfaction as the process is really about flavour recognition. Its perception depends on all the properties of the familiar food – vision, taste, texture and smell – being integrated to help conjure the characteristic odour:

> We are harnessing the brain to take over and bypass the injury and to use information from memory and so will work with individuals' most familiar foods, to tailor each trial for each one. The hard part for us now is recruiting enough subjects.

26

A New Olfactory Future

I talk to my parents in Sydney most weekends and our chats helped break the boredom of the long lockdowns in London at a time when Australians still had their freedoms, thanks to early and tough border closures. It was only then that I learned that my father, Paolo, had lost his sense of smell many years before and, with hindsight, thought it had disappeared a good decade before he received a diagnosis of Parkinson's disease. At the time this ignited a new anxiety for me, so when my olfactory system began to recover a few months later, every fragrance that returned amplified my sense of relief and gratitude.

The realisation that my father's olfactory loss had not been seen as a red flag by the GP at the time bothered and angered me a little too. In my year-long journey to understand the human olfactory system, I'd read some rigorous and indisputable research on the prevalence of smell loss in Parkinsonism – more than 95 per cent of patients report it before any other symptoms, often many years in advance of being diagnosed.[1] Professor Antje Haehner, a German specialist in chemosensory loss and neurodegenerative disease and lead author of one of these major studies, told me that solid evidence is also accumulating to show that the sooner Parkinson's patients are placed on appropriate medication, even before motor symptoms appear, the better their long-term health outcomes and quality of life. She herself had had the chance to observe male twins, her patients, who had both been diagnosed early with Parkinson's. One chose to commence medication immediately while the other did not. 'Over time, there were great differences in their symptoms and also in their quality of life,' she said.

My father's disease has been managed very well for many years: he himself often says how grateful he is for the neurological care he has received. But that early, unheeded note of warning from his nose only served as another stark reminder to me that our sense of smell has been dangerously underrated – and even cruelly mistrusted – for too long.

※

The implications of anosmia are vast. Not only does the sense of smell create scaffolding for fundamental chemosensory learning and communication between humans almost from conception but it continues to influence our emotional and psychological well-being throughout our lives. Its disappearance can occasionally have sinister origins: Parkinson's is not the only neurodegenerative disease associated with this symptom. More than a third of multiple sclerosis patients suffer smell loss[2] and, according to Professor Haehner, it is also associated with 85 to 90 per cent of patients suffering Alzheimer's disease: 'Deficits in smell identification can often predict decline or clinical conversion from mild cognitive impairment to the dementia of Alzheimer's.'

It seems a no-brainer then – pardon the pun – that smell testing should be incorporated into routine health checks as part of a measure of overall physiological and emotional well-being, perhaps even at the level of the GP's surgery, particularly if a patient presents with a smell or taste concern. The NHS in the UK and many other national health systems worldwide offer a battery of tests, including liver function, blood sugars and blood pressure, as part of preventative health policies for those aged fifty and over. Despite growing volumes of knowledge about the diagnostic and predictive benefits of smell function (not just for neurodegenerative diseases but for others with known links including depression, dystonia[3] and schizophrenia[4]) the incorporation of smell testing has been widely ignored or even resisted.

Part of the problem, as is often the case, is cost.[5] The single use UPSIT (University of Pennsylvania Smell Identification Test) costs around £20 per patient while a full set of the Sniffin' Sticks, which measure threshold and discrimination as well as identification, would set a clinic back £800 for each one. While this offers a much lower per patient cost, clinicians must be trained in their use and they take precious face-to-face time to administer. At a time when national health systems are grappling with ever-dwindling limited resources, longer consultations and extra per patient cost is always going to be resisted.

But perhaps this is where Covid might represent a silver lining for long-term health policy-makers: at no time in modern history has the olfactory system been studied so intensely by so many. At the time of writing, medRxiv and bioRxiv, the pre-print servers for research papers in the health sciences and biology, had more than 1,500 publications lined up awaiting peer review, nearly five times the number produced in the year before Covid arrived.

The library of knowledge is growing exponentially too as opportunities to study the brains of patients suffering olfactory disturbances has exploded. While the earliest days of the pandemic meant that most imaging and radiological studies focused on acute single cases, time and the sheer number of patients with mild respiratory symptoms but marked olfactory and gustatory disturbances has provided clinicians and scientists with thousands of brains and noses to image study. The UK Biobank, one of the world's largest biomedical databases, containing the genetic and health information of more than half a million people, had already scanned the brains of more than 40,000 participants before Covid. In the summer of 2021, a group of Oxford neuroscientists published an intriguing pre-print of a study in which they had invited nearly 800 of these participants back, carefully choosing similar ages, ethnicities and other variants. Of these, half had tested positive for Covid and reported mild or no symptoms and the balance were controls.[6]

This kind of study, with matched cases to their controls, offers a rare and premium standard in epidemiology and allowed researchers to examine more than 2,300 different brain measurements, a mind-boggling experiment. These differences were then whittled down to the 300 or so brain measurements that the scientists felt could plausibly be associated with Covid damage. This mix of data analysis and direct physiological study meant they were able to identify significant reductions in grey-matter thickness and volume in the olfactory bulb parts of the brain related to memory and smell – just as has been seen in patients with some neurodegenerative diseases.

Alarming as this may seem for the many millions of us who have been struck by Covid-induced anosmia, it's important to remember that subtle brain changes don't necessarily imply disease or that they're permanent: the researchers themselves made very clear that while they interpret their findings to show the irrefutable harm inflicted by the virus as it enters the nose and affects the brain, it might also suggest that changes to the olfactory regions are a consequence of the loss of taste and smell – not necessarily the cause of it. (Remember how our olfactory bulbs show a loss of volume when we lose our sense of smell – and an increase as we recover – another example of the 'use it or lose it' principle at its vivid best.) When I read and digested the Oxford study, I was ecstatic that I now understood enough about the olfactory system to understand this important, if subtle, difference and not fall into a panic!

The development of new smell tests appropriate to different age groups and cultures and that can be administered quickly, inexpensively and even at home has been on the drawing board of many more European and US clinics and universities. But Covid has added new impetus and energy to this work too and many more nations have been working towards this end. In the UK, researchers at Queen Mary University of London have recently developed a capsule-based smell test that requires the patient to crush it between their fingers and remove a taste strip to release the smell. A score based on how many smells the patient identifies correctly can then be sent to the GP for further diagnostics. Its lead researcher, Dr Ahmed Ismail, says the capsule test is quick, can assist not just in flagging possible neurodegenerative diseases but can also be applied to Covid diagnosis: 'Being non-invasive and less stressful, it has benefits over the nose swab in diagnosing Covid. This is an advantage for testing children in particular as they are horrified by nose swabs and this test can be done at home.'

During some of my earliest conversations with scientists involved in olfactory research as the Covid pandemic took hold, it was clear that they very quickly recognised the invaluable, unexpected opportunities to unearth new knowledge in the wake of a concurrent global anosmia epidemic. Kicked out of their laboratories during the interminable lockdowns, they formed collaborative networks first to find out just how the novel virus infected the olfactory systems and later to explore new and creative ways to understand more about the mechanisms of smell. Equally importantly, the thousands of Covid patients who had first-hand experience of smell loss and distortion could now describe what happened to them along the road to recovery. Their descriptions and collaboration continue to offer real, contemporary, qualitative data that will further close the gap between researchers working in laboratories and the rest of the population.

Dr Federica Genovese, a young Italian neuroscientist working at the Monell Chemical Senses Center in Philadelphia, was one of the very first I spoke to and her sense of energy and excitement was infectious even then as she described the way her colleagues the world over from this relatively small, niche area – from senior professorial level to young post-doctoral students – had thrown themselves into trying to 'connect the dots':

How the olfactory community came together in this huge collaborative effort . . . I've never seen that in my life. Many of us felt a strong sense of duty to put aside rivalry. We weren't allowed in the labs and we had to work in other ways, work differently and not just sit at home going crazy. We [in olfactory research] are a small area but I think finally it has also helped the medical community to realise just how smell and taste have not been understood enough, not taken care of enough in patients, smell tests not taught so that any basic generalist doctor could do it.

Bob Datta agrees:

One of the key things that has emerged in the wake of Covid is that we have all learned that it is impossible to go it alone. Clinicians, basic scientists, epidemiologists, scientists concerned with human physiology, chemosensory scientists, everyone involved in human taste and smell at global scale knows we need to interact at many levels. That has been one of the most exciting and gratifying things . . . if you look at the author list on our paper, it spans expertise from across the globe. It required the collaboration of many people across the field, some that we'd normally never have collaborated with and yet we did, all of us sharing a common goal. It is a kind of historic culture change.

For physicians and researchers such as Professor Hummel and forty-one professorial and senior colleagues working in some of the world's most prestigious university hospital otorhinolaryngology departments, the new, global spotlight on the sense of smell represents a vindication of decades of work – even if they would never be so ungracious as to describe it this way. Specialists from Harvard Medical School in Boston to University College in London to Konkuk University in Seoul, South Korea, to the Surgery Hospital in Istanbul among a host of others became signatories to a detailed manifesto and call to arms to olfactory clinicians and researchers worldwide, imploring them to 'adopt a common language' to improve the methodological quality, consistency and – I love this word – 'generalisability' of work in their field. Published in the journal *Rhinology*, the thirty-page paper sets out a roadmap to shake up the way clinicians and researchers manage patients, requiring that they take complaints of suspected olfactory loss seriously and offer full examinations of the head and neck, including nasal endoscopy. The paper warned against clinicians offering subjective assessments of smell loss in isolation and pushed for the use of reliable and validated tests for at least two smell examinations, threshold and identification or discrimination.

As I thought about their united and spirited counsel and what I had learned from my own anosmia, it seemed incredible there should even be a need for such a diagnostic protocol to be proposed and put on paper.

Think about it, if your eyes suddenly lost their potency to see and the world became blurred, difficult to navigate and frightening, your GP would immediately order a battery of tests, from functional and ophthalmic through to brain imaging if necessary to diagnose the problem. And yet here we are in the twenty-first century and it took a pandemic to highlight the need for equivalent, standardised diagnostic responses to the loss of smell.

§

For Datta and many of his colleagues working at the frontline of global olfactory research and discovery, Covid is a game-changer, one with profound and, it is to be hoped, some beneficial long-term consequences.

We humans, he observes, are so profoundly visual and tactile that for too long we have thought of these two senses as the most relevant to our daily lives, to how we interact with others and understand our world. But the olfactory system is ancient, was the first of our sensory systems to evolve and is hard-wired into memory and emotion.

> When you look at an object, it takes about ten synapses for information to get from the back of your eyeball to your retina to some part of your brain that drives an emotion. But it's just one synapse away, from your nose to your bulb and into your amygdala. There is this incredibly intimate inter-action between your sense of smell and the parts of your brain that tell you you're okay, you're centred in the world and you understand what is going on around you . . . I think the dislocation that has happened to millions of people as a consequence of their loss of smell has really highlighted the importance of understanding how the system works and developing therapies for when it's broken. The truth is that because it has been such an under-appreciated sense,

we have only scratched the surface of understanding how the 800 or so chemicals that make up the head space of the coffee I'm drinking now are somehow synthesised by my brain into this unitary sense that lets me know my morning is going to be okay. We are just at the beginnings of understanding that process and there is so much left to discover.

I asked the eminent scientist why he thought smell has been the poor cousin in research labs for so long. Is it traditional lack of resources with the majority of funding channelled into sight and hearing, or is it the sheer complexity of the olfactory system that makes unravelling its mysteries so difficult?

I think it's probably both. The reality is that the vast majority of resources do go into hearing and sight. It makes perfect sense: audition and verbal communication are critical to our identities as humans. But that has had the unfortunate consequence of maybe making it seem like olfaction and taste are not that important and I think we're learning they are. For some people, loss of smell causes a shift in psychological state that can lead to real disease, to depression – it is a well-known risk factor. I really hope psychiatrists, psychologists and clinicians who see olfaction patients work together to manage that. We have never had a pandemic that has caused multiple millions of people to lose their sense of smell for a long period of time. As far as we know, this has never happened before and we are going to have to deal with the consequences.

Because, you know, they *are* coming.

Epilogue

As I put the finishing touches to this book and look back over the journey, I want to give hope to the tens of thousands of people who are still struggling with anosmia and parosmia. Don't give up. Keep smell training and reminding your nose and brain of smells that meant something to you. Exercise your nose, even if it is frustrating, because that old adage 'use it or lose it' is true for the fifth sense too.

My diagnostic tests, conducted in Dresden with the Sniffin' Sticks under the watchful eye of Professor Hummel, illustrated with precision what I had felt instinctively about my recovery. My sense of smell had returned after more than a year and the threshold tests – which determine the lowest concentration of an odorant I can detect – confirmed that I was back in the realm of what is normal for women in my age group. But when it came to identifying familiar smells or registering the difference between, say, apple and cinnamon, banana and bubble-gum, I faltered. My body had done its work regenerating and recovering after the Covid virus ravaged the olfactory epithelium but my ability to identify odorants and not simply perceive a familiarity remains below par. Based on my results the advice was clear: daily practice and exercise of odour-identification powers is imperative.

Regaining the sense of smell is about more than just, well, smelling. We must all spend time remembering fragrances, imagining them, testing ourselves daily, using, exercising – and challenging – our entire olfactory system.

We must continue to do this even at times when it feels hopeless – and especially when we think our sense of smell is returning. If you are lucky enough to recover from anosmia, the relief and happiness at being able to smell anything at all can also lead to complacency. Just as stroke or brain-injury survivors have to strive to find ways for their brains to compensate for lost functions, we need to do the same for our sense of smell. I had been content to train my nose with my personal array of perfumes and did so every day – but it wasn't enough. The neural pathways that were regenerating also needed more practice in making those important connections correctly and with different odorants. Smell training, like exercise, needs not just to become a daily routine but one that progresses, finds new personal challenges and even sets future goals.

Medical science has astounded us during the pandemic. Large trials of Vitamin A – identified way back in the 1960s as beneficial in helping the regeneration of damaged nasal mucosa – are under way at the University of East Anglia for use by Covid anosmia sufferers. Drugs such as cerebrolysin, used to aid neuroplasticity and neuro-regeneration in stroke and traumatic brain-injury patients, are also being re-examined for their potential for olfactory recovery. Smell training is also being tested again; what was a relatively unknown technique is now being added to more and more olfactory clinicians' arsenal. Our sense of smell has been thrust into the public spotlight in an unprecedented way, an unforeseen consequence of a pandemic that, tragically, has stolen the lives of millions. If there is a silver lining to this terrible chapter in modern human history, it is that it has forced a re-evaluation of our sense of smell, not just for its importance to our quality of life but as a powerful sentinel and hitherto unsung surveillance system that when properly read can tell us so much about our physical and mental health.

·

Exactly eighteen months after becoming anosmic, I had an experience that would have been inexplicable before embarking on my journey to understand the fifth sense. We were on holiday in Puglia, in the south of Italy, and had ventured out into the white-washed streets of a little medieval town called Locorotondo for a sunset aperitif when the church bells began to ring. As we walked up the limestone cobbles towards the town's main gate, a procession bearing a black-robed Virgin Mary – *la Madonna del'Addolorata* – emerged from the church doors, her life-size effigy and golden platform carried on the backs of four, female parishioners. A youngish, handsome Jesuit led the procession, flanked by two older diocesan priests in flowing white vestments, while another parishioner carrying an incense-burner on long chains pushed onwards through the growing crowd.

As the plume of fragrant smoke curled, swirled, expanded and entered my nostrils, my eyes filled with unexpected tears and my throat choked with emotion. In an instant, the smouldering frankincense and myrrh had transported me back to childhood and attending Mass with my grandmother. We returned to Italy from Australia every two years and those summers, back in the bosom of grandparents and cousins, had instilled a lifetime's longing and nostalgia. I am not religious and even as a young child questioned the Catholic faith but, somehow, the rituals and smells of those glorious, innocent days of childhood had imprinted into my brain and here they were, detonated inside me via my newly functional nose. I am sure that if Robert had not witnessed the tears, visible and undeniable, I'd have relegated the moment to imagination.

Never could I have had a more powerful reminder of the joy of the olfactory sense, its profound and enduring mysteries – and what may be missed when it malfunctions.

Nasal cavity

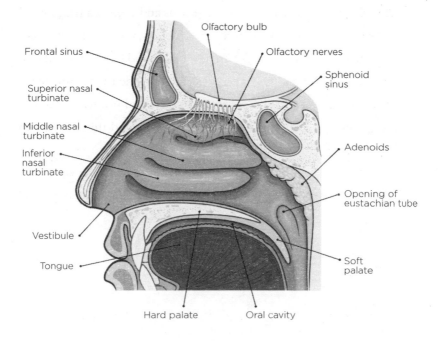

Olfactory bulb

Frontal sinus

Olfactory nerves

Superior nasal turbinate

Sphenoid sinus

Middle nasal turbinate

Inferior nasal turbinate

Adenoids

Opening of eustachian tube

Vestibule

Tongue

Soft palate

Hard palate

Oral cavity

Olfactory system

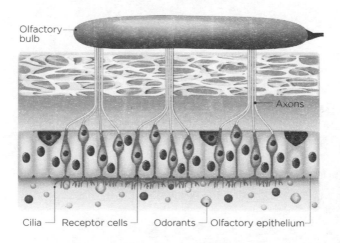

Olfactory bulb

Axons

Cilia

Receptor cells

Odorants

Olfactory epithelium

Acknowledgements

This book was conceived of loss – and yet so much has been gained giving it life!

First and foremost, thank you to my co-author and husband, Robert, whose writing mantra 'Stop talking about it, just do it' meant we did exactly that; a team in life and love.

Delving into the world of our endlessly complex, precious and remarkable fifth sense has been a challenge and a joy; embarking on the journey to document this unique moment in human scientific history, a privilege.

However, writing this book would not have been possible without the extraordinary intellectual generosity of the olfactory research community worldwide. They represent myriad disciplines – neuroscience, chemistry, philosophy, anthropology, medicine – and each and every one opened their prodigious minds (and sometimes also their laboratories) to us. I don't need to list you all one by one, your voices are inside these pages. But special thanks to Professors Thomas Hummel and Barry Smith, Drs Jane Parker, Duika Burges Watson (and soon-to-be PhD, Aidan Kirkwood for his eleventh-hour support).

A heartfelt thanks also to *The Australian* newspaper editors who first saw the story's potential; Doug Young at Pew Literary in London for helping re-imagine it into a book; and our UK publisher, Olivia Bays, and her team at Elliott & Thompson for its painless delivery.

Last but not least, our gratitude goes to Chrissi Kelly, tireless patient advocate and founder of anosmia charity AbScent, who has helped us articulate the experiences of – and give hope to – the many thousands who are still grieving the loss of their sense of smell.

References

1: The Story of O(lfaction)

1. 'Ancient bacteria alive and well', *Trends in Microbiology*, vol. 9, no. 1 (January 2001), p. 12; doi.org/10.1016/S0966-842X(00)01926-0
2. R. Nijland and Professor J. G. Burgess, 'Bacterial olfaction', *Biotechnology Journal*, vol. 5, no. 9 (September 2010), pp. 974–7; doi.org/10.1002/biot.201000174
3. A. S. Barwich, *Smellosophy: What the Nose Tells the Mind* (Cambridge, MA: Harvard University Press, 2020)

2: The Scent of Daffodils

1. C. Wordsworth, *Memoirs of William Wordsworth, Poet-laureate D.C.L.* (London: Edward Moxon, 1851)
2. R. Southey, *Life and Correspondence of Robert Southey*, vol. 1 (1822), p. 63
3. R. Southey, *The Life and Correspondence of Robert Southey*, vol. III, edited by C. C. Southey (London: Longmans, 1850), p. 313; accessed via www.lordbyron.org/monograph.php?doc=RoSouth.1849&select=III.XVI
4. R. J. Littman and M. L. Littman, 'Galen and the Antonine plague', *American Journal of Philology*, vol. 94, no. 3 (1973), pp. 243–55; www.jstor.org/stable/293979
5. K. Robinson, *The Sense of Smell in the Middle Ages: A Source of Certainty* (Abingdon: Routledge, 2019)
6. Wellcome collection, wellcomecollection.org/articles/XamCsxAAACAAqWIm
7. M. Lucenet, 'La peste, fléau majeur' (Université de Paris, 1994), quoted and translated in Michel Tibayrenc (ed.), *Encyclopedia of Infectious Diseases: Modern Methodologies* (Hoboken, NJ: Wiley-Liss, 2007) p. 680

Further reading:

Feigel, L. (ed.), *A Nosegay: A literary journey from the Fragrant to the Fetid* (London: Old Street Publishing, 2006)

Wordsworth, W., 'Musings Near Acquapendente', Memorials of a Tour in Italy, 1837 (London: Edward Moxon, 1842)

Letters between Wilson and Wordsworth, 1802, held in the Wordsworth Trust

3: From Fragrances Foul

1. https://archeologie.culture.fr/lascaux/en/father-andre-glory-1906-1966
2. D. Ackerman, *A Natural History of the Senses* (New York: Random House, 1990), p. 60
3. M. Macleod, 'Eau de BO: The allure of sweat', *New Scientist*, 9 May 2012; www.newscientist.com/article/mg21428641-600-eau-de-bo-the-allure-of-sweat/
4. E. de Feydeau, *A Scented Palace: The Secret History of Marie Antoinette's Perfumer* (London: I. B. Tauris, 2006)
5. J. Hogg, *London as It Is: Being a series of observations on the health, habits and amusements of its people* (London: John Macrone, 1837)
6. A. Corbin, *The Foul and the Fragrant: Odour and the French Social Imagination* (New York: Berg, 1986), p. 4
7. ibid.
8. D. S. Barnes, *The Great Stink of Paris and the Nineteenth-Century Struggle against Filth and Germs* (Baltimore: Johns Hopkins University Press, 2006), pp. 17, 20, 237
9. C. Classen, D. Howes and A. Synnott, *Aroma: The Cultural History of Smell* (Abingdon: Routledge, 1994), p. 81
10. G. W. S. Piesse, *Piesse's Art of Perfumery* (London: Piesse and Ludin, 1891), cited in Classen et al., *Aroma*

Further reading:

Trueman, J., *The Romantic Story of Scent* (New York: Doubleday, 1975)

Aftel, M., *Essence and Alchemy: A book of Perfume* (London: Bloomsbury, 2001)

4: Scent and Sensibility

1. W. H. Perkin, 'On the artificial production of coumarin and formation of its homologues', *Journal of the Chemical Society*, vol. 21 (1868), pp. 53–63; doi.org/10.1039/JS8682100053
2. L. Turin and T. Sanchez, *Perfume: The A–Z Guide* (London: Profile Books, 2008), p. 35
3. Z. Gorvett, 'The delicious flavour with a toxic secret', BBC, 20 June 2017; www.bbc.com/future/article/20170620-the-delicious-flavour-with-a-toxic-secret
4. H. Melville, *Moby Dick* (London: Longman, 2009), p. 407

5. Genesis 9:3, King James Bible; www.kingjamesbibleonline.org/Genesis-9-3/
6. Plato, *The Republic*, http://classics.mit.edu/Plato/republic.10.ix.html
7. D. M. Stoddart, *The Scented Ape* (London: Cambridge University Press, 1990), p. 6
8. Stanford Encyclopedia of Philosophy, 2002; https://plato.stanford.edu/entries/condillac/
9. I. Kant, *Anthropology from a Pragmatic Point of View* [1798] (Cambridge, Cambridge University Press, 2006), pp. 50–51
10. C. Darwin, *The Descent of Man* (London: John Murray, 1871)
11. P. Broca, 'Recherches sur les centres olfactifs', *Revue d'Anthropologie*, 2ème série, tome II (1879), pp. 385–455
12. J. P. McGann, 'Poor Human Olfaction is a nineteenth-century myth', *Science*, 12 May 2017; www.ncbi.nlm.nih.gov/pmc/articles/PMC5512720/
13. A. Gilbert, *What the Nose Knows: The Science of Scent in Everyday Life* (Crown, 2008; ebook, Synthetics, 2014)
14. H. Ellis, 'Sexual Selection in Man: Touch, Smell, Hearing, and Vision' Part 1, in *Studies of Psychology of Sex*, vol. 2 (Philadelphia: F. A. Davis, 1905), cited in Barwich, *Smellosophy*, p. 37
15. N. Elias, *The Civilising Process* (Oxford: Blackwell, 1977–82), vol. 2, p. 297
16. M. Smith, *Sensory History*, cited in M. S. R. Jenner, 'Follow Your Nose? Smell, Smelling and Their Histories', *The American Historical Review*, no. 2 (April 2011), pp. 335–51; www.jstor.org/stable/23307699
17. J. Zhang and D. M. Webb, 'Evolutionary deterioration of the vomeronasal pheromone transduction pathway in catarrhine primates', *Proceedings of the National Academy of Sciences*, vol. 100, no. 14 (July 2003), pp. 8337–41; doi.org/10.1073/pnas.1331721100
18. D. M. Stoddart, *Adam's Nose and the Making of Humankind* (London: Imperial College Press, 2015)

5: Beauty without Smell

1. M. Tafalla, 'A World without the Olfactory Dimension', *The Anatomical Record*, vol. 296, no. 9 (2013), pp. 1287–96; doi.org/10.1002/ar.22734
2. M. Proust, *In Search of Lost Time* (London: Penguin Classics, 2003)
3. M. Tafalla, 'Smell and Anosmia in the Aesthetic Appreciation of Gardens', *Contemporary Aesthetics*, vol. 12 (2014), pp 19–27; hdl.handle.net/2027/spo.7523862.0012.019
4. M. Tafalla, 'Anosmic Aesthetics', *Estetika, the European Journal of Aesthetics*, vol. 50, no. 1 (2013), pp. 53–80; doi.org/10.33134/eeja.103
5. L. Lundqvist, *A World Without Smells* (Createspace, 2017)

6: Mapping the Nose

1. O. Walusinski, 'Joseph Hippolyte Cloquet (1787–1840) – Physiology of smell: Portrait of a pioneer', *Clinical and Translational Neuroscience* (2018), cited in M. Cobb, *Smell: A Very Short Introduction* (Oxford, Oxford University Press, 2020)

2. E. A. McC. Gamble, 'The applicability of Weber's Law to smell', *American Journal of Psychology*, vol. 10, no. 1 (1898), pp. 82–142; doi.org/10.2307/1412679

3. L. B. Buck and R. Axel, 'A novel multigene family may encode odorant receptors: A molecular basis for odorant recognition', *Cell*, vol. 65 (1991), pp. 175–87; doi.org/10.1016/0092-8674(91)90418-x

7: The Taste of Rotting Water

1. D. Hare, *Beat the Devil: A Covid Monologue* (London: Faber & Faber, 2020)

2. All quotes sourced from the AbScent Facebook group, used with permission.

3. J. K. Parker, C. E. Kelly, B. C. Smith, A. F. Kirkwood, C. Hopkins and S. Gane, 'Patients' perspectives on qualitative olfactory dysfunction: Thematic analysis of social media posts', *JMIR Formative Research*, vol. 5, no. 12 (2021); doi.org/10.2196/29086

4. D. L. Burges Watson, M. Campbell, C. Hopkins, B. Smith, C. Kelly et al., 'Altered smell and taste: Anosmia, parosmia and the impact of long Covid-19', *PLoS One*, vol. 16, no. 9 (2021); doi.org/10.1371/journal.pone.0256998

5. D. L. Burges Watson et al., 'Altered eating: A definition and framework for assessment and intervention', *BMC Nutrition*, vol. 4, no. 14 (2018); doi.org/10.1186/s40795-018-0221-3

Further reading:

Keller, A. and Malaspina, D., 'Hidden consequences of olfactory dysfunction: a patient report series', *BMC Ear Nose Throat Disorders*, vol. 13, no. 8 (2013); doi.org/10.1186/1472-6815-13-8

10: Science on the Scent

1. D. H. Brann, T. Tsukahara, C. Weinreb, M. Lipovsek, K. Van den Berge, B. Gong, R. Chance, I. C. Macaulay, H. J. Chou, R. B. Fletcher, D. Das, K. Street, H. R. de Bezieux, Y. G. Choi, D. Risso, S. Dudoit, E. Purdom, J. Mill, R. A. Hachem, H. Matsunami, D. W. Logan, B. J. Goldstein, M. S. Grubb, J. Ngai and S. R. Datta, 'Non-neuronal expression of SARS-CoV-2 entry genes in the olfactory system suggests mechanisms underlying COVID-19-associated anosmia', *Science Advances*, vol. 6, no. 31 (2020); doi.org/10.1126/sciadv.abc5801

2. M. Zazhytska, A. Kodra, D. A. Hoagland, J. F. Fullard, H. Shayya, A. Omer, S. Firestein, Q. Gong, P. D. Canoll, J. E. Goldman et al., 'Non-cell autonomous

disruption of nuclear architecture as a potential cause of COVID-19 induced anosmia', *Cell* (February 2022); doi.org/10.1016/j.cell.2022.01.024

Further reading:

Nagashima, A. and Touhara, K., 'Enzymatic conversion of odorants in nasal mucus affects olfactory glomerular activation patterns and odor perception', *Journal of Neuroscience*, vol. 30, no. 48 (December 2010), pp. 16391–98; doi. org/10.1523/JNEUROSCI.2527-10.2010

11: AbScentia

1. S. H. Bagheri, A. Asghari, M. Farhadi, A. R. Shamshiri, A. Kabir, S. K. Kamrava, M. Jalessi, A. Mohebbi, R. Alizadeh, A. A. Honarmand, B. Ghalehbaghi, and A. Salimi, 'Coincidence of Covid-19 epidemic and olfactory dysfunction outbreak', *Medical Journal of the Islamic Republic of Iran*, vol. 34, no. 62 (2020); www.medrxiv.org/content/10.1101/2020.03.23.20041889v1

2. M. Roberts, 'Coronavirus: Are loss of smell and taste key symptoms?', BBC News, 1 April 2020; www.bbc.co.uk/news/health-52111606

12: A Political Stink

1. R. C. Gerkin et al., 'Recent smell loss is the best predictor of Covid-19 among individuals with recent respiratory symptoms', *Chemical Senses*, vol. 46 (January 2021); doi.org/10.1093/chemse/bjaa081

13: Smell Warp

1. O. Perl, E. Mishor, A. Ravia, I. Ravreby and N. Sobel, 'Are humans constantly but subconsciously smelling themselves?', *Philosophical Transactions of the Royal Society Series B*, vol. 375, no. 1800 (2020); https://royalsocietypublishing.org/doi/10.1098/rstb.2019.0372

2. C. Hopkins, P. Surda, L. A. Vaira, J. Lechien, M. Safarian, S. Saussez and N. Kumar, 'Six months follow up of self reported loss of smell during the Covid-19 pandemic', *Rhinology*, vol. 59, no. 1 (2021), pp. 26–31; doi. org/10.4193/Rhin20.544

3. ibid.

4. J. K. Parker, C. E. Kelly and S. B. Gane, 'Molecular Mechanism of Parosmia', medRxiv (2021); doi.org/10.1101/2021.02.05.21251085

15: My Designated Nose

1. C. Song and B. E. Leonard, 'The olfactory bulbectomised rat as a model of depression', *Neuroscience and Biobehavioral Reviews*, vol. 29, nos. 4–5 (2005), pp. 627–47; doi.org/10.1016/j.neubiorev.2005.03.010

16: The Devil Inside

1. P. Süskind, *Perfume: The Story of a Murderer* (London: Penguin, 1985)
2. Song and Leonard, 'The olfactory bulbectomised rat as a model of depression'

17: The Grandfather of Olfaction

1. G. Kobal and C. Hummel, 'Cerebral chemosensory evoked potentials elicited by chemical stimulation of the human olfactory and respiratory nasal mucosa', *Electroencephalography and Clinical Neurophysiology*, vol. 71, no. 4 (1988), pp. 241–50; doi.org/10.1016/0168-5597(88)90023-8
2. R. S. Herz, J. Eliassen, S. Beland and T. Souza, 'Neuroimaging evidence for the emotional potency of odour-evoked memory', *Neuropsychologia*, vol. 42, no. 4 (2004), pp. 371–8; doi.org/10.1016/j.neuropsychologia.2003.08.009
3. R. Herz, *The Scent of Desire* (New York: Harper Collins, 2007)
4. A. Arshamian, E. Iannilli, J. C. Gerber, J. Willander, J. Persson, H. S. Seo, T. Hummel and M. Larsson, 'The functional neuroanatomy of odour-evoked autobiographical memories cued by odours and words', *Neuropsychologia*, vol. 51, no. 1 (2013), pp. 123–31; doi.org/10.1016/j.neuropsychologia.2012.10.023
5. T. Hummel and I. Croy, 'Olfaction as a marker of depression', *Journal of Neurology*, vol. 264, no. 4 (2017), pp. 631–8; doi.org/10.1007/s00415-016-8227-8
6. Q. Li, D. Yang, et al., 'Reduced amount of olfactory receptor neurons in the rat model of depression', *Neuroscience Letters*, vol. 603 (2015), pp. 48–54; doi.org/10.1016/j.neulet.2015.07.007
7. A. Cavazzana, S. C. Poletti, C. Guducu, M. Larsson and T. Hummel, 'Electro-olfactogram responses before and after aversive olfactory conditioning in humans', *Neuroscience*, vol. 373 (2018), pp. 199–206; doi.org/10.1016/j.neuroscience.2018.01.025

18: The Chemistry of Love

1. C. M. Drea, 'Design, delivery and perception of condition-dependent chemical signals in strepsirrhine primates: implications for human olfactory communication', *Philosophical Transactions of the Royal Society Series B*, vol. 375 (2020); doi.org/10.1098/rstb.2019.0264
2. J. Porter, B. Craven, R. M. Khan, S. J. Chang, I. Kang, B. Judkewicz, J. Volpe, G. Settles and N. Sobel, 'Mechanisms of scent-tracking in humans', *Nature Neuroscience*, vol. 10, no. 1 (2007), pp. 27–29; doi.org/10.1038/nn1819
3. C. Ferdenzi, S. R. Ortegón, S. Delplanque, N. Baldovini and M. Bensafi, 'Interdisciplinary challenges for elucidating human olfactory attractiveness', *Philosophical Transactions of the Royal Society Series B*, vol. 375 (2020); doi.org/10.1098/rstb.2019.0268

4. B. Schaal, L. Marlier and R. Soussignan, 'Human Foetuses learn odours from their pregnant mother', *Chemical Senses*, vol. 25, no. 6 (2000), pp. 729–37; doi. org/10.1093/chemse/25.6.729

5. B. Schaal, L. Marlier and R. Soussignan, 'Olfactory function in the human fetus: evidence from selective neonatal responsiveness to the odour of amniotic fluid', *Behavioral Neuroscience*, vol. 112 (1998), pp. 1438–49; doi.org/10.1 037/0735-7044.112.6.1438

Further reading:

Almagor, U., 'The cycle and stagnation of smells: Pastoralists-fishermen relationships in an East African society', *RES: Anthropology and Aesthetics*, vol. 13 (1987), pp. 106–121; doi.org/10.1086/RESv13n1ms20166765

Classen, C., 'The odor of the other: olfactory symbolism and cultural categories', *Ethos*, vol. 20, no. 20 (1992), pp. 133–66; doi.org/10.1525/eth. 1992.20.2.02a00010

Majid, A. and Kruspe, N., 'Hunter-gatherer olfaction is special', *Current Biology*, vol. 28, no. 3 (2018), pp. 409–413; doi.org/10.1016/j.cub.2017.12.014

Mennella, J. A., Jagnow, C. P. and Beauchamp, G. K., 'Prenatal and postnatal flavor learning by human infants', *Pediatrics*, vol. 107, no. 6 (2001); doi.org/10.1542/ peds.107.6.e88

Pandya, V., 'Movement and space: Andamanese cartography', *American Ethnologist*, vol. 17, no. 4 (1990), pp. 775–797; doi.org/10.1525/ae.1990.17.4. 02a00100

19: Smell is the Scaffolding

1. C. Darwin, 'A biographical sketch of an infant', *Mind*, vol. 2, no. 7 (1877), pp. 285–94; doi.org/10.1093/mind/os-2.7.285

2. A. Macfarlane, 'Olfaction in the development of social preferences in the human neonate', Parent-Infant Interaction (Ciba Foundation Symposium 33), vol. 33 (1975), pp. 103–17; doi.org/10.1002/9780470720158.ch7

3. R. H. Porter, J. W. Makin, L. B. Davis and K. M. Christensen, 'An assessment of the salient olfactory environment of formula-fed infants', *Physiology & Behaviour*, vol. 50, no. 5 (1991), pp. 907–11; doi.org/10.1016/0031-9384(91) 90413-I

4. A. M. Widström, G. Lilja, P. Aaltomaa-Michalias, A. Dahllöf, M. Lintula and E. Nissen, 'Newborn behaviour to locate the breast when skin-to-skin: a possible method for enabling early self-regulation', *Acta Paediatrica*, vol. 100, no. 1 (2011), pp. 79–85; doi.org/10.1111/j.1651-2227.2010.01983.x

5. S. Doucet, R. Soussignan, P. Sagot and B. Schaal, 'An overlooked aspect of the human breast: areolar glands in relation with breastfeeding pattern, neonatal

weight gain, and the dynamics of lactation', *Early Human Development*, vol. 88, no. 2 (2012), pp. 119–28; doi.org/10.1016/j.earlhumdev.2011.07.020

6. B. Schaal, S. Doucet, R. Soussignan, M. Klaey-Tassone, B. Patris and K. Durand, 'The human mammary odour factor: variability and regularities in sources and functions', in C. Buesching (ed.), *Chemical Signals in Vertebrates*, vol. 14 (Cham, Switzerland: Springer, 2019), pp. 118–138; doi.org/10.1007/978-3-030-17616-7_10

7. B. Schaal, G. Coureaud, D. Langlois, C. Ginies, E. Sémon and G. Perrier, 'Chemical and behavioural characterization of the rabbit mammary pheromone', *Nature*, vol. 424 (2003), pp. 68–72; doi.org/10.1038/nature01739

8. S. Doucet, R. Soussignan, P. Sagot and B. Schaal, 'The "smellscape" of mother's breast: effects of odour masking and selective unmasking on neonatal arousal, oral, and visual responses', *Developmental Psychobiology*, vol. 49, no. 2 (2007), pp. 129–38; doi.org/10.1002/dev.20210. PMID: 17299785

9. K. Durand, J. Y. Baudouin, D. J. Lewkowicz, N. Goubet and B. Schaal, 'Eye-catching odours: Olfaction elicits sustained gazing to faces and eyes in 4-month-old infants', *PLoS One*, vol. 8, no. 8 (2013); doi.org/10.1371/journal.pone.0070677

20: The Smell of Fear

1. J. Williams, C. Stönner, J. Wicker, N. Krauter, B. Derstroff, E. Bourtsoukidis et al., 'Cinema audiences reproducibly vary the chemical composition of air during films, by broadcasting scene specific emissions on breath', *Scientific Reports*, vol. 6, 25464 (2016); doi.org/10.1038/srep25464

2. J. H. B. de Groot, P. A. Kirk and J. A. Gottfried, 'Titrating the smell of fear: Initial evidence for dose-invariant behavioral, physiological, and neural responses', *Psychological Science*, vol. 32, no. 4 (2021), pp. 558–72; doi.org/10.1177/0956797620970548

3. J. G. Goldman, 'What our perspiration reveals about us', BBC, 4 August 2015; www.bbc.com/future/article/20150803-what-our-perspiration-reveals-about-us

Further reading:
Wicker, J., Krauter, N., Derstroff, B., Stönner, C., Bourtsoukidis, E., Klüpfel, T., et al., 'Cinema data mining: The smell of fear' in *Proceedings of the 21st ACM SIGKDD International Conference on Knowledge Discovery and Data Mining* (New York: ACM, 2015), pp. 1295–1304; doi.org/10.1145/2578726.2578744

21: Speaking of Smells

1. D. Lynott et al., 'The Lancaster sensorimotor norms: multidimensional measures of perceptual and action strength for 40,000 English words',

Behavior Research Methods, vol. 52 (2020), pp. 1271–91; doi.org/10.3758/s13428-019-01316-z

2. O. Koblet and R. S. Purves, 'From online texts to Landscape Character Assessment: collecting and analysing first-person landscape perception computationally', *Landscape Urban Planning*, vol. 197 (2020); doi.org/10.1016/j.landurbplan.2020.103757

3. A. Majid, 'Human olfaction at the intersection of language, culture, and biology', *Trends in Cognitive Sciences*, vol. 25, no. 2 (2021), pp. 111–23; doi.org/10.1016/j.tics.2020.11.005

4. F. U. Jönsson and M. J. Olsson, 'Olfactory Metacognition', *Chemical Senses*, vol. 28, no. 7 (2003), pp. 651–8; doi.org/10.1093/chemse/bjg058

5. L. Meteyard, B. Bahrami and G. Vigliocco, 'Motion Detection and Motion Verbs: Language Affects Low-Level Visual Perception', *Psychological Science*, vol. 18, no. 11 (2007), pp. 1007–13; doi.org/10.1111/j.1467-9280.2007.02016.x

6. J. K. Olofsson and J. A. Gottfried, 'The muted sense: neurocognitive limitations of olfactory language', *Trends in Cognitive Sciences*, vol. 19, no. 6 (2015); doi.org/10.1016/j.tics.2015.04.007

7. Majid, 'Human Olfaction at the Intersection of Language, Culture, and Biology'

8. A. Majid et al., 'Differential coding of perception in the world's languages', *Proceedings of the National Academy of Sciences of the United States of America*, vol. 115, no. 45 (6 November 2018), pp. 11369–76; www.jstor.org/stable/e26563143

9. A. Majid and N. Burenhult, 'Odours are expressible in language, as long as you speak the right language', *Cognition*, vol. 130, no. 2 (2014), pp. 266–70; doi.org/10.1016/j.cognition.2013.11.004

10. A. Majid and N. Kruspe, 'Hunter gatherer olfaction is special', *Current Biology*, vol. 28, no. 3 (2018), pp. 409–13; doi.org/10.1016/j.cub.2017.12.014

11. A. Arshamian, P. Manko and A. Majid, 'Limitations in odour simulation may originate from differential sensory embodiment', *Philosophical Transactions of the Royal Society Series B*, vol. 375 (2020); doi.org/10.1098/rstb.2019.0273

12. R. J. Stevenson and M. K. Mahmut, 'The accessibility of semantic knowledge for odours that can and cannot be named', *Quarterly Journal of Experimental Psychology*, vol. 66, no. 7 (2013), pp. 1414–31; doi.org/10.1080/17470218.2012.753097

22: Parfum Eau de Poo

1. F. Grabenhorst, E. T. Rolls and C. Margot, 'A hedonically complex odour mixture produces an attentional capture effect in the brain', *NeuroImage*, vol. 55, no. 2 (2011), pp. 832–43; doi.org/10.1016/j.neuroimage.2010.12.023

23: Smelly Stories of Art and Industry

1. J. Card, 'Tips for boosting productivity with good office design', *Guardian*, 23 January 2014; www.theguardian.com/small-business-network/2014/jan/23/productivity-office-design

24: Tip of the Iceberg

1. Pamphlet by A. G. Bell, 1914 'Discovery and Invention', reprinted from *National Geographic Magazine*, June 1914, by the National Geographic Society; downloaded from Library of Congress
2. J. del Mármol, M. A. Yedlin and V. Ruta, 'The structural basis of odorant recognition in insect olfactory receptors', *Nature*, vol. 597 (August 2021), pp. 126–31; doi.org/10.1038/s41586-021-03794-8
3. J. K. Taubenberger, 'The origin and virulence of the 1918 "Spanish" influenza virus', *Proceedings of the American Philosophical Society*, vol. 150, no. 1 (2006), pp. 86–112
4. R. T. Ravenholt and W. H. Foege, '1918 influenza, encephalitis lethargica, parkinsonism', *Lancet*, vol. 2 (1982), pp. 860–4; doi.org/10.1016/s0140-6736(82)90820-0

Further reading:

Vijgen, L., Keyaerts, E., Moës, E., et al., 'Complete genomic sequence of human coronavirus OC43: molecular clock analysis suggests a relatively recent zoonotic coronavirus transmission event', *Journal of Virology*, vol. 79, no. 3 (2005), pp. 1595–604; doi.org/10.1128/JVI.79.3.1595-1604.2005

Brüssow, H. and Brüssow, L., 'Clinical evidence that the pandemic from 1889 to 1891 commonly called the Russian flu might have been an earlier coronavirus pandemic', *Microbial Biotechnology*, vol. 14, no. 5 (2021), pp. 1860–70; doi. org/10.1111/1751-7915.13889

25: Hope in the Time of Anosmia

1. D. G. Laing and G. W. Francis, 'The capacity of humans to identify odours in mixtures', *Physiology & Behavior*, vol. 46, no. 5 (1989), pp. 809–14; doi.org/10.1016/0031-9384(89)90041-3
2. D. G. Laing, A. Epps and A. L. Jinks, 'Chemosensory loss during a traumatic brain injury suggests a central pathway for the rehabilitation of anosmia', *Chemical Senses*, vol. 46 (2021); doi.org/10.1093/chemse/bjab016
3. C. Zelano, A. Mohanty and J. A. Gottfried, 'Olfactory predictive codes and stimulus templates in piriform cortex', *Neuron*, vol. 72, no. 1 (2011), pp. 178–87; doi.org/10.1016/j.neuron.2011.08.010

26: A New Olfactory Future

1. A. Haehner, S. Boesveldt, H. W. Berendse, A. Mackay-Sim, J. Fleischmann, P. A. Silburn, A. N. Johnston, G. D. Mellick, B. Herting, H. Reichmann and T. Hummel, 'Prevalence of smell loss in Parkinson's disease – a multicenter study', *Parkinsonism & Related Disorders*, vol. 15, no. 7 (2009), pp. 490–4; doi. org/10.1016/j.parkreldis.2008.12.005

2. A. Carotenuto, T. Costabile, M. Moccia, F. Falco, M. R. Scala, C. V. Russo, F. Saccà, A. De Rosa, R. Lanzillo and V. Brescia Morra, 'Olfactory function and cognition in relapsing, remitting and secondary-progressive multiple sclerosis', *Multiple Sclerosis and Related Disorders*, vol. 27 (2019), pp. 1–6; doi. org/10.1016/j.msard.2018.09.024

3. T. Herr, J. Gamain, R. Fleischmann, et al., 'Olfaction as a marker for dystonia: Background, current state and directions', *Brain Sciences*, vol. 10, no. 10 (2020), p. 727; doi.org/10.3390/brainsci10100727

4. S. F. Dingfelder, 'In brief: Schizophrenia may be characterized by unique smell deficits', *Monitor on Psychology*, vol. 35, no. 7 (2004); www.apa.org/monitor/jun04/schizo

5. L. Langstaff, A. Clark, M. Salam et al., 'Cultural adaptation and validity of the Sniffin' Sticks psychophysical test for the UK setting', *Chemosensory Perception*, vol. 14 (2021), pp. 102–8; doi.org/10.1007/s12078-021-09287-2

6. G. Douaud, S. Lee, F. Alfaro-Almagro, C. Arthofer, C. Wang, F. Lange, J. L. R. Andersson, L. Griffanti, E. Duff, S. Jbabdi, B. Taschler, A. Winkler, T. E. Nichols, R. Collins, P. M. Matthews, N. Allen, K. L. Miller and S. M. Smith, 'Brain imaging before and after COVID-19 in UK Biobank', medRxiv (2021); doi.org/10.1101/2021.06.11.21258690

Index